Radiology Cases for the MRCP

Vincent Williamson DMRD, FRCR

Consultant Radiologist
Dept of Radiology
Arrowe Park Hospital, Upton
Wirral, Merseyside

Debra King FRCP

Consultant Physician in geriatric medicine
Department of Medicine for the elderly
Wirral Hospital
Arrowe Park Road, Upton
Wirral, Merseyside

 W. B. SAUNDERS COMPANY LTD

Edinburgh • London • New York • Philadelphia • Sydney • Toronto 1999

W. B. SAUNDERS
An imprint of Harcourt Brace and Company Limited

© Harcourt Brace & Company Limited 1999

 is a registered trade mark of Harcourt Brace and Company Limited

First published 1999

ISBN 0702023639

British Library Cataloguing in Publication Data
A catalogue record for this book is available from the British Library.

Library of Congress Cataloging in Publication Data
A catalog record for this book is available from the Library of Congress.

Medical knowledge is constantly changing. As new information becomes available, changes in treatment, procedures, equipment and the use of drugs become necessary. The authors and the publishers have, as far as it is possible, taken care to ensure that the information given in this text is accurate and up to date. However, readers are strongly advised to confirm that the information, especially with regard to drug usage, complies with current legislation and standards of practice.

Printed in China

Dedication

To my parents, wife and children, Clare and Emma.

V. C. W.

Acknowledgements

We would like to thank Mrs Susan Stewart for her support and expert typing of the manuscript. We are also grateful to the Department of Medical Photography at Arrowe Park Hospital for assistance with the illustrations.

Contents

'Apparatuses are cleverer than man and anyone who mishandles apparatus is my enemy.'

W.K. Röntgen (1845–1923), German physicist.

Wilhelm Konrad Röntgen was a professor of physics and director of the Institute of Physics in Würzburg. In 1895 he discovered X-rays and the science of radiology was born. He was awarded the Nobel prize in physics for his discovery in 1901. In 1900 he was appointed professor of physics at the University of Munich, where he remained until his retirement in 1920. He died of carcinoma of the rectum in 1923.

Introduction

There is a close relationship between radiologist and physician; both work synergistically to enable a diagnosis to be made. More commonly nowadays radiologists also perform therapeutic radiological procedures such as abscess drainage under X-ray control, insertion of oesophageal/ angiographic stents, to name but two. It is important that the physician has knowledge of the necessity for radiological investigations and the possibility of therapeutic radiological procedures. MRCP candidates are therefore required to have a basic knowledge of radiological interpretation as it applies to clinical practice. Any radiological tests may be included as part of the written examination, mainly in the photographic section, but films/scans etc. may also be shown to a candidate during the discussion of a case in the clinical examination. As well as chest radiograph interpretation, films which the candidate may be shown include: CT scans, MRI scans, barium examinations, angiograms, isotope bone scans and lung scans, among others. It is important to have some understanding of the quality of a film and of the pitfalls of interpretation. These are described in the interpretation section of this book. The cases that follow are typical clinical cases which may be part of the photographic section of the examination or may require interpretation during a short or long clinical case. There is often a clue to the answer in the initial few statements given which provide clinical pointers. Each case is followed by the kind of discussion which may be required in the clinical/oral section of the examination. Clinical symptoms and signs are included as far as possible in each case. The main discussion points are included but candidates who require more detail are advised to consult a reference text.

Film interpretation

CHEST RADIOGRAPH

Before you can interpret a chest radiograph, or indeed any radiograph, you have to be sure that it was taken in the correct manner. If it was not, this can cause you to 'see' pathology that is not there or miss pathology that is there.

Factors to consider on a chest radiograph

1. *Is the whole area of interest on the film?* The costophrenic angles are the commonest area to be missed off, especially in large patients.
2. *Was the patient straight when the film was taken?* This is assessed by looking at the medial ends of the clavicles relative to the spine (vertebral body and its spinous process).

   ● Straight (Fig. 1a). Clavicle to spinous process distance the same on both sides.

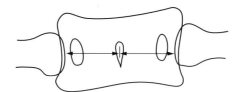

Fig. 1a

   ● Rotated (Fig. 1b).

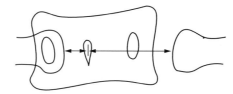

Fig. 1b

   If the patient has a thoracic scoliosis then the radiographer may not be able to get the patient straight. A rotated film results in:
   — Difference in transradiancy (degree of blackness) of the two lungs. The lung on the side to which the patient is turned is blacker. This can be mistaken for abnormal shadowing in the other lung.
   — Apparent difference in volume of the two lungs.
   — Apparent widening of the mediastinum.
   — Apparent cardiac enlargement as the heart lies obliquely.
   — Obscuration of the hila. A tumour or lymphadenopathy may be missed.

4

3. *Was the correct exposure used?* A correctly exposed film should allow you to see good detail in the lungs (vessels, any nodules or other shadowing) and also detail at the left base behind the heart. If the exposure is too high, lung detail is blacked out. If the exposure is too low then:
— The heart and breast shadows obscure the lung bases.
— There is apparent shadowing in both lungs. As a result, acute pulmonary oedema can be diagnosed in a normal chest.

Having ensured that your film is not deceiving you because of technical factors you only have to spot, and interpret, the pathology!

WHAT TO LOOK FOR

1. The cardiac shadow

(a) Heart size

A frontal chest film can be taken in one of two ways, anteroposterior (AP) or posteroanterior (PA). With an AP projection the film is behind the patient and the X-ray machine in front. The beam therefore passes through the chest from anterior to posterior (Fig. 2).

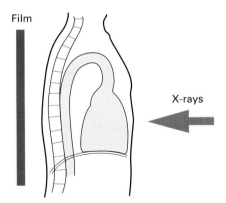

Film

X-rays

Fig. 2

A PA projection is the reverse of this situation. The importance of all this is that the X-ray beam is diverging from its source in the X-ray set. Therefore the further something is from the film the more it is magnified (Fig. 3).

5

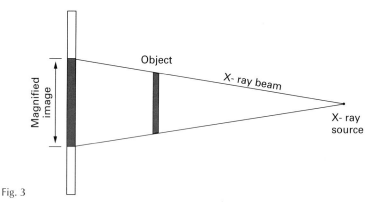

Fig. 3

As the heart is an anterior structure, it is less magnified if the film is against the front of the chest (PA projection). A PA film is therefore ideal. With an AP film the degree of magnification varies with the size of the patient. As a result most films are performed PA. An AP may be performed, however, with very sick patients who cannot be moved from their bed/trolley/wheelchair. Assessment of cardiac size is based on the PA film. The diameter of the heart is compared to the internal diameter of the chest (from the inner rib surface to inner rib surface). If the heart is not enlarged this cardiothoracic ratio (CTR) is less than 50%. Be sure, however, that the film is not rotated (see above) and that you measure only the heart and not any pericardial fat pads that may be present. On a well exposed film these are seen to be of lesser density than the heart. They are usually triangular in shape and lie in the costophrenic angles (Fig. 4).

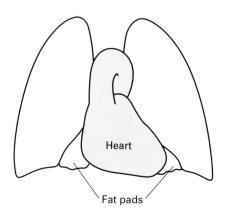

Fig. 4

On the AP film cardiac size is harder to assess. If the CTR is less than 50% then the heart is obviously not enlarged. If the heart is huge then it is obviously enlarged. Between these two situations one cannot be sure.

(b) Heart size

Congenital heart disease is beyond the scope of a short account like this. There are, however, some characteristic shapes to look out for in acquired heart disease.

- **Pericardial effusion.** The heart is enlarged and of a globular shape such as one might expect with a bag full of fluid.
- **Left atrial enlargement (mitral heart).** The left atrium lies just below the carina. As the atrium enlarges the carinal angle is splayed with elevation of the left main bronchus. The enlarged atrium also increases the density of the cardiac shadow centrally and it can be seen as a double shadow on the right side of the heart. The left atrial appendage is seen as a bulge on the left heart border (Fig. 5).

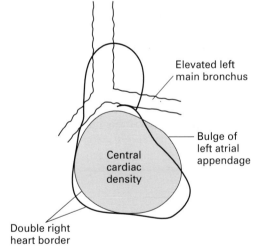

Elevated left main bronchus

Bulge of left atrial appendage

Central cardiac density

Double right heart border

Fig. 5

As the left atrium lies posteriorly when enlarged, it is seen to bulge posteriorly on the lateral radiograph (Fig. 6).

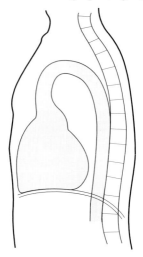

Fig. 6

(c) Cardiac orientation

- Dextrocardia may be an isolated finding, part of complete situs inversus, or related to some syndromes (e.g. Kartagener's), but beware of incorrectly labelled films or the film being put up the wrong way round.
- Right-sided aortic arch may be part of dextrocardia or may occur with normal cardiac orientation. Again there are associations, such as Fallot's tetralogy and its variants, truncus arteriosus, and corrected transposition of the great arteries.

2. Pulmonary vessels

As well as the pulmonary plethora or oligaemia seen in some congenital cardiac anomalies, one needs to look out for:

(a) Pulmonary venous congestion seen in cardiac failure
Upper lobe blood diversion can be a feature but is an unreliable sign. A supine radiograph invalidates the sign (as the upper lobes are not upper-most). Also, pre-existing basal lung disease may cause it, or upper lobe disease prevent it from occurring.

(b) Pulmonary arterial hypertension
Large central pulmonary arteries with peripheral cut off.

8

3. Pulmonary shadowing

This is often divided into *alveolar* and *interstitial* shadowing. These can be useful descriptions in ordering one's thoughts to reach a diagnosis. They do not reliably reflect the pathological distribution of disease.

Alveolar shadowing is homogenous shadowing that may contain an air bronchogram (air containing airways shown up by the opacification of the surrounding lung). This form of shadowing can be due to filling of the air spaces by:

● Pus (pneumonia)
● Fluid (pulmonary oedema)
● Blood (pulmonary haemorrhage)
● Tumour (alveolar cell carcinoma).

Interstitial shadowing may be reticular (linear), nodular, or a combination of the two (reticulonodular). It may reflect interstitial pulmonary oedema, fibrosis or other reflections of interstitial (diffuse lung) disease.

The same pathology may cause both, for example cardiac failure. As left atrial pressure rises, first upper lobe blood diversion occurs, then interstitial pulmonary oedema (Kerley lines), then alveolar oedema.

With diffuse lung disease the distribution is as important as the pattern in reaching a diagnosis:

Mainly basal disease

● Fibrosing alveolitis, either cryptogenic or associated with collagen vascular disease
● Fibrosis related to some drugs
● Asbestosis. Look for evidence of pleural plaques and pleural thickening.

Mainly upper lobe disease

● TB (look out for calcification)
● Sarcoidosis (mid and upper zones)
● Extrinsic allergic alveolitis (chronic fibrotic stage)
● Allergic bronchopulmonary aspergillosis (look for bronchiectasis as well as fibrosis)
● Ankylosing spondylitis (look for changes in the spine)
● Post radiotherapy (likely to be unilateral unless mediastinal, in which case the lung fibrosis parallels the mediastinum)

- Progressive massive fibrosis (pneumoconiosis). The fibrotic masses mop up the nodules of pneumoconiosis and migrate towards the hila
- Cystic fibrosis (children and young adults).

Unilateral disease

Lymphangitis carcinomatosa (linear shadowing), (look for hilar carcinoma or lymphadenopathy).

Nodular shadowing is seen in:

- Sarcoidosis (hard, well defined nodules)
- Extrinsic allergic alveolitis, subacute pattern (soft, ill defined nodules)
- Metastases
- Infection (including miliary TB, fungal and viral pneumonia)
- Coal workers' pneumoconiosis and silicosis.

4. Lung masses

- Solitary or multiple. Multiple lesions suggest metastases or arteriovenous malformations in hereditary haemorrhagic telangectasia
- Size
- Shape: round, lobulated, spiculated. This is of limited use. Metastases are usually round but a primary lung carcinoma may also be round. Spiculation is seen in lung cancer but also in fibrosis
- Site (which lobe?)
- Associated features. Bony destruction, adjacent to chest wall or mediastinum, pleural effusion, mediastinal or hilar lymphadenopathy.

5. Lobar collapse or consolidation

Contours such as the heart borders can be seen because aerated lung lies adjacent to soft tissue density. If the lung aeration is lost, so is the contour. Which borders are lost gives a clue to the lobe involved (e.g. right middle lobe – right heart border; lingular segment – left heart border; lower lobes – hemidiaphragms).

Different lobes collapse in a different pattern.

● Right upper lobe collapse; horizontal fissure swings up and medially. The trachea deviated to the side of the collapse (Fig. 7).

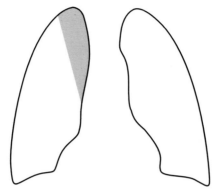

Fig. 7

● Right middle lobe (Fig. 8); loss of the right heart border on the frontal film. Collapse seen on lateral film.

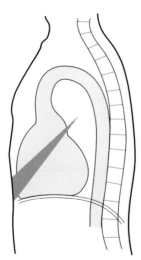

Fig. 8

● Right lower lobe (Fig. 9).

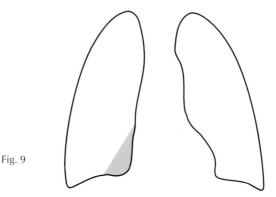

Fig. 9

● Left upper lobe collapse (Fig. 10): on the frontal view there is no well defined lower border as there is no horizontal fissure on the left. The shadowing just gradually fades out down the lung.

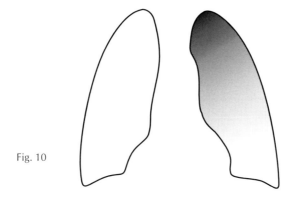

Fig. 10

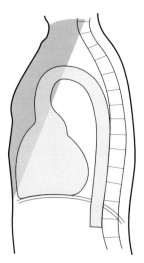

Fig. 11

On the lateral view the lobe is seen to have collapsed anteriorly (Fig. 11).

- Left lower lobe collapse (Fig. 12). Triangular shadow behind the heart.

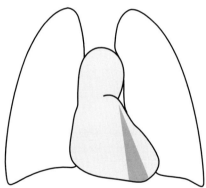

Fig. 12

Collapse can also result in shift of the mediastinal structures, hilum and hemidiaphragm and the ribs look closer together on the site of collapse.

6. Pleural space

(a) Pleural effusion

Opacification, possibly of the whole hemithorax. If the effusion is large then there is mediastinal shift to the other side, unless there is underlying lung collapse. A meniscus appearance can be seen on the film if the patient was erect, but not when there is complete white-out. (An opaque hemithorax is also seen in collapse of a whole lung or following pneumonectomy. Mediastinal shift and surgical clips should give clues to the latter.) Also, there is no meniscus seen if the patient is supine as the fluid lies posteriorly, producing hazy shadowing.

(b) Pneumothorax
A black rim is seen with a visible lung edge and no lung markings beyond this. A hydropneumothorax results in a horizontal air fluid level on an erect film.

(c) Pleural or subpleural mass (Figs 13a and 13b)
A lung mass may reach or even invade the pleura (Fig. 13b) but its angle with the pleural surface is typically different from one arising in the pleura or subpleural space (Fig. 13a). Such masses have a longer point of contact with the pleural surface and taper gradually.

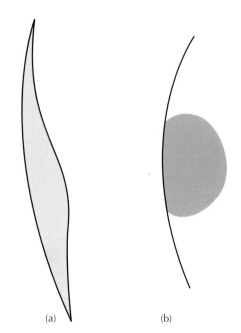

Fig. 13   (a)   (b)

A pleural mass may be a plaque or thickening, loculated pleural fluid, a pleural fibroma, mesothelioma or metastasis. Subpleural masses include rib metastases or myeloma deposits that have soft tissue extension outside the bone.

7. Mediastinum

A mediastinal mass may arise in any of the structures found there. In making a differential diagnosis it is useful to localize the mass with respect to the anterior, middle or posterior mediastinum. Germ cell tumours, thyroid and thymic masses are typically anteriorly placed. Neurogenic and oesophageal tumours lie more posteriorly. Lymphadenopathy can occur at any site. Calcification or fat within a mass may suggest a germ cell tumour.

8. Bones

Metastases, like myeloma, usually result in bone destruction (lytic lesions). Bony metastases from some primary sites can be sclerotic (denser than normal), however. The commonest primary sites for sclerotic deposits are prostatic carcinoma (in men) and breast carcinoma (in women). Other bony lesions such as rib destruction by a Pancoast's tumour or fractures should also be looked for.

9. Subdiaphragmatic air

This is most commonly due to perforation of a duodenal ulcer. It is well shown on an erect chest film, but be careful not to mistake air in the stomach or bowel for a perforation.

ABDOMINAL RADIOGRAPH

1. Bowel gas and free gas

The visible gas should be within the stomach or bowel, but it can be seen outside the gastrointestinal tract in cases of perforation or intra-abdominal abscess. An abscess may be seen as a rounded air collection or speckled in appearance (usually they are not visible on plain films, however, and require ultrasound or CT to demonstrate them). Perforation is most easily seen as subdiaphragmatic air on an erect chest film. On a supine abdominal film its presence can be revealed when one can see both sides of the bowel wall outlined by air (rather than just the inner side).

Bowel obstruction is suggested by dilatation proximally, which should suggest the site of the problem. However, an ileus also causes bowel dilatation as does pseudo-obstruction. The colon can normally appear quite dilated in the elderly.

Bowel wall oedema can be seen as a pattern called thumbprinting. This is seen in inflammatory bowel disease, ischaemia etc.

2. Calcification

Calcification may be seen in a large number of situations in the abdomen:

- Phleboliths. These are of no significance and are usually pelvic in location. They are often multiple and appear small, round and frequently with a central lucency
- Arterial (look out for an aortic aneurysm)
- Gall stones (only 10% calcify)
- Renal and ureteric stones (90% calcify)
- Bladder stones
- Mesenteric lymph nodes. A common normal finding in older patients
- Pancreatic calcification in chronic pancreatitis. Speckled calcification in the site and shape of the pancreas
- Renal and colonic carcinomas may calcify, as may some renal cysts
- Ovarian carcinomas and teratomas
- Uterine fibroids.

3. Bones

The bones should be examined for evidence of metastases or other bony pathology such as sacroileitis in patients with inflammatory bowel disease.

4. Soft tissue masses

Soft tissue masses may be seen on a plain film as can hepatomegaly or splenomegaly.

CT OF THE BRAIN

Computed tomography employs X-ray sources and detectors set in a rotating ring to obtain axial slices through the region of interest. The degree to which each tissue in the image attenuates the beam is given a numerical value between +1000 and −1000. This scale is centred on water at a value of 0. The less the beam attenuation, the lower the number. These numerical values are displayed as a grey scale from black up to white (i.e. the more attenuation of the beam the whiter the tissue appears). The picture displayed is made up of dots (called pixels) which are a two-dimensional representation of a small volume of tissue (called a voxel). As the full range from +1000 to –1000 is too great to be displayed on an image with any worthwhile contrast, a range is chosen to show the tissue of interest to best advantage. For the brain one would centre the image around +35 and have the grey scale cover a window width of 80. All tissue of values above the displayed range would appear as white and all those below the range as black (in this case fat and air would appear featureless and black, calcification or bone would be featureless and white).

THE MAIN INDICATIONS FOR CT OF THE BRAIN

1. Severe head injury

To show any skull fracture the window levels of the image would need to be altered to show bone. The brain is the main concern, however. The brain may just appear swollen or there may be evidence of a haematoma. Fresh intracranial blood appears white on the window settings used for the brain. Over the next 2–3 weeks it gradually becomes the same value as brain tissue and then darker than brain. Blood may be seen within the brain, in the ventricles and basal cisterns, or in the subdural or extradural spaces. The difference between a subdural and an extradural haematoma can be determined from their shape. The **extradural** space between the skull vault and the dura is quite tight and a bleed here is confined to a bi-convex shape (Fig. 14a).

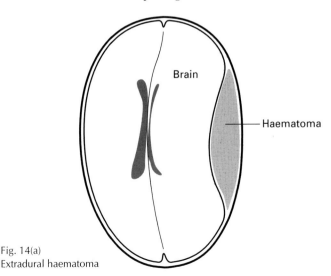

Fig. 14(a)
Extradural haematoma

An extradural haematoma is usually in the temporal region and results from damage to the middle meningeal artery. A **subdural haematoma** results from tearing of bridging veins at the brain surface. As the subdural space is less tight the haematoma can spread out in the space between the arachnoid and dura producing a shape which conforms to the brain surface (Fig. 14b).

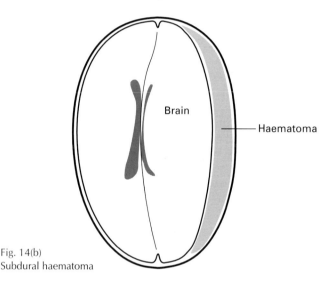

Fig. 14(b)
Subdural haematoma

Both have mass effect producing effacement of the sulci, compression of the ventricles and midline shift to the other side. Fresh white blood in the ventricles and other CSF spaces is easily seen relative to the normal (black) CSF.

2. Subarachnoid haemorrhage

Again fresh blood appears white on CT images of the brain. In subarachnoid haemorrhage it may be seen in the basal cisterns, sylvian fissures, sulci over the brain surface and in the ventricular system. Sometimes some blood is also seen within the brain substance. The distribution of the blood may give a clue to the site of berry aneurysm that caused it, but often does not. The aneurysm itself is usually not visible on the acute CT scan.

3. Stroke

A stroke may be an infarct or bleed. The latter is of course white (possibly with a little surrounding oedema which is dark grey in colour). An infarct appears as dark grey. It too may have mass effect acutely due to oedema. While an infarct may be visible on CT within 24 hours, it is at its maximum visibility at 3–5 days when oedema is at its greatest. Despite a typical stroke history, however, CT sometimes shows no abnormality as the infarct responsible is beyond the resolution of the scan.

4. Tumour

The three commonest intracranial tumours in adults are metastases, glioma and meningioma. All three produce mass effect and can have associated oedema (though this is less in the case of meningiomas). They all enhance (become whiter) following intravenous contrast medium as there is no blood – brain barrier in the tumour. Meningiomas may be of higher attenuation than normal brain even before contrast injection. They may also contain calcification (again of high attenuation and therefore appearing white), as may gliomas. Meningiomas arise from a meningeal surface whereas gliomas and metastases arise within the brain (although they may, of course, reach the brain surface). Multiple lesions suggest metastases, though gliomas or meningiomas can be multiple. Gliomas are often cystic with an enhancing rim and metastases may also show some necrosis.

5. Intracranial abscess

An abscess is seen as a ring structure (with enhancement of the wall after intravenous contrast) and surrounding oedema. Like tumours they have mass effect. Prior to abscess formation there is cerebritis which is seen as oedema, though there may be contrast enhancement within it.

THE INTRAVENOUS UROGRAM

The intravenous urogram (IVU) used to be the standard investigation of the urinary tract, but now ultrasound has replaced it in many cases. An IVU is still the investigation of choice in renal colic and to demonstrate transitional cell carcinoma of the urothelium.

Ultrasound is preferable to demonstrate renal cell carcinoma and in imaging patients with prostatism or urinary tract infection.

The IVU starts with a control film prior to the injection of intravenous contrast medium. This film will show any calcification including calculi (90% of renal calculi calcify). Oblique views may be needed to confirm whether a possible calculus is really renal or just projected over the kidney (if it is renal it will move with the kidney on the other projection).

The contrast is then injected and an immediate film of the kidneys obtained to show the renal substance during the nephrogram phase. Assuming that there is no contraindication (e.g. renal colic or other abdominal pain, aortic aneurysm or recent abdominal surgery), a compression band is then applied across the lower abdomen to distend the pelvicalceal systems adequately. Another view of the kidneys is then done at 5–10 minutes after injection to show the collecting systems. It is on this image that one looks for filling defects such as a transitional cell carcinoma. Tomography (producing coronal slices) can be done at this stage, if needed, to show detail if there is overlying bowel. The compression is then released and a full length abdominal film obtained to show the ureters, looking for filling defects or their relationship to any possible calculus. Full and empty bladder films are also taken, to exclude a filling defect and confirm full emptying on micturition. A common incidental finding in the pelvis is the presence of phleboliths. These are of calcific density and can be mistaken for calculi in the lower ureter. Helpful distinguishing features are that phleboliths tend to be round with a central lucency while ureteric calculi are usually slightly elongated. Phleboliths can also be shown to be outside the ureters on post contrast films of the IVU series. Another possible trap is mistaking an area of arterial wall calcification for a stone. Again the IVU, by showing the ureters, demonstrates such calcification to be outside the urinary tract. Both renal and bladder tumours can calcify, as occasionally can the walls of simple renal cysts. If a bladder tumour is found it is important to look closely in the pelvicaliceal systems and ureters as transitional cell carcinomas can be multiple. In renal colic one can expect to see hydronephrosis and ureteric dilatation above the level of the stone. Excretion of the contrast is often delayed and late films are then needed to demonstrate the site of obstruction.

BARIUM AND OTHER CONTRAST STUDIES OF THE GASTROINTESTINAL TRACT

Barium sulphate alone or double contrast with air is the standard contrast medium for the gastrointestinal tract (GIT). It can demonstrate the whole GIT from hypopharynx to the rectum, but not in a single examination. There are four basic examinations:

Barium swallow

This is used to demonstrate a cause for dysphagia. It should include the hypopharynx, oesophagus and stomach. If the site of dysphagia is low then the hypopharynx examination can be omitted but the reverse is not true as sometimes the level of dysphagia can seem to be higher than the lesion. Also, cricopharyngeal spasm, one cause of high dysphagia, is often secondary to gastro-oesophageal reflux. The hypopharynx and upper oesophagus are examined using either a rapid film sequence on camera or videofluoroscopy. The abnormalities that may be seen include a post cricoid web, a pharyngeal pouch, benign or malignant oesophageal strictures, gastro-oesophageal reflux, with or without a hiatus hernia or ulceration.

Barium meal

An examination of the oesophagus, stomach and duodenum. Usually a smooth muscle relaxant (hyoscine butylbromide or glucagon) is given intravenously to improve the images. The main indications are gastro-oesophageal reflux, peptic ulcer disease and carcinoma. Endoscopy has reduced the level of demand for barium meals. It has the advantage of allowing a biopsy to be performed. This is especially important when a gastric ulcer is seen as they can be malignant. A malignant duodenal ulcer would be very rare (as is small bowel carcinoma).

Barium small bowel study

This can be performed as a 'follow through' examination or as a small bowel enema. The former involves the patient drinking a large amount of barium sulphate. In the small bowel enema a tube is passed via the nose down into the duodenum and the barium sulphate is then run in through this. This may be followed by air, water or methylcellulose to provide a double contrast examination. In most cases, however, the follow through type of examination is sufficient and is less unpleasant for the patient. Whichever one one does, it is purely an examination of the small bowel. A 'barium meal and follow through' cannot be performed as this represents two examinations at the same time. They involve a different technique, including the concentration of barium sulphate solution used. If one were to attempt to do both at a single sitting one would just end up with two poor examinations rather than anything useful. Crohn's disease is the commonest indication for a small bowel study. Small bowel lymphoma can occur, as can carcinoma, but this is rare. All of these can produce stricturing with ulceration.

Barium enema

An examination of the large bowel. Smooth muscle relaxants are usually given and barium sulphate solution, followed by air, is introduced. The commonest indications are diverticular disease, suspected large bowel carcinoma or inflammatory bowel disease. It is an unpleasant and invasive test and elderly patients can often find it difficult to retain the enema. Oral ferrous sulphate should be discontinued 7 days prior to the examination as it coats the colonic mucosa and mucosal lesions can be missed.

Water soluble contrast medium

These are needed when a leak is suspected, such as at an anastomotic site or a perforation. Barium sulphate must not be used if there is a risk of a leak into the mediastinum or peritoneal cavity. Gastografin can be used to demonstrate perforations, but caution is needed in the upper gastro-intestinal tract as aspiration into the lungs can produce severe pulmonary oedema. The contrast media that are used intravenously in the IVU or CT are safe in any situation, however. None of these alternative contrast media produces as good mucosal detail as barium sulphate. They are used only when the use of barium is not considered to be safe.

NUCLEAR MEDICINE

Most diagnostic imaging gives anatomical information but nuclear medicine gives a functional picture. A radioistope is linked to a carrier molecule that targets the tissue to be studied. The anatomical resolution is poor, but taken with other imaging these examinations are of great use. The commonest examinations performed in a district general hospital setting are the bone scan and ventilation and perfusion lung scan. In the bone scan ^{99m}Tc (technetium) is linked to a bone seeking agent MDP (methylene diphosphonate). This is taken up in normal bone but areas of increased bone turnover show up as high uptake lesions. The appearance is non-specific, however, and the assessment must include the clinical picture and the plain radiographs of the abnormal areas. Reasons for increased uptake include fractures, metastases, osteomyelitis and Paget's disease.

The ventilation/perfusion lung scan is still the standard investigation of suspected pulmonary embolism. One is looking for perfusion defects with normal ventilation. However, interpretation is not straightforward and the scan is expressed as normal, low, intermediate/indeterminate or high probability of pulmonary embolism. The biggest problem is in the patients with chronic obstructive pulmonary disease where the scan result falls into the indeterminate classification. About 40% of scans are classed as intermediate/indeterminate probability and 33% of these will have a pulmonary embolism (PE). Clinical probability of a PE is also taken into account, but further investigation with pulmonary arterio-graphy, spinal CT angiography or Doppler ultrasound or venography of the lower limbs to look for deep venous thrombosis (the likely source of the PE) is needed in difficult cases. The perfusion images are obtained by injecting macroaggregates or microspheres labelled with ^{99m}Tc. Ventilation can be with xenon or krypton gas or ^{99m}Tc DTPA (Diethylene Triamine Penta-acetic Acid) aerosols. The latter are easier logistically but the images are inferior.

Cases

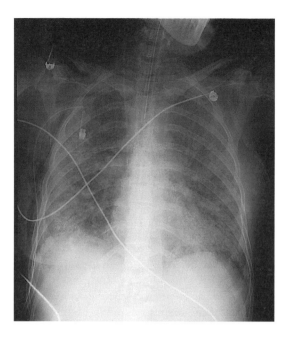

Questions

This 56-year-old lady was under the care of the haematologists prior to this acute admission. She is now very ill on the intensive care unit. Her blood results on admission were:

- Hb 13.4 g/dl
- MCV 85.6 fl
- RBC 4.58 × 10^{12}/l
- Platelets 382 × 10^9/l
- WBC 43.4 × 10^9/l (73% neutrophils, 5% lymphocytes, 5% monocytes, 4% basophils, 1% metamyelocytes, 9% myelocytes, 1% promyelocytes, 2% blasts).

On transfer to ITU her blood results were:

- Hb 8.2 g/dl
- RBC 2.76 × 10^{12}/l
- Platelets 173 × 10^9/l
- WBC 21.8 × 10^9/l (96.4% neutrophils).

a. Name four abnormalities on her chest X-ray.
b. What was her pre-existing haematological condition?

Answers

a. The film shows an endotracheal tube and central venous line in satisfactory positions. The endotracheal tube should, as here, be well above the carina. There is a right-sided chest drain in situ with surgical emphysema in the chest wall. The patient has had a pneumothorax, either as a complication of mechanical ventilation, or insertion of the central venous line. There are also cardiac monitor leads present. The heart size is normal. The widespread pulmonary shadowing is of the alveolar type as seen in infection, pulmonary oedema, pulmonary haemorrhage, or occasionally tumour.

b. Chronic myeloid leukaemia.

Discussion

In haematological malignancies such lung shadowing as is seen here can be due to direct malignant involvement of the lungs, pulmonary haemorrhage, a reaction to the chemotherapy (e.g. pulmonary oedema) or infection (the patient being immunosuppressed both by the disease and by the treatment). The usual treatment for the chronic phase of CML is busulphan. The pulmonary adverse effects of this can be fibrosis, diffuse alveolar damage or pulmonary vasculitis. Pulmonary toxicity may develop within a few months of commencing treatment or take several years. Ultimately CML transforms into a frankly malignant condition as seen here with myelocytic precursor cells and blasts in the peripheral blood with a fall in red cell count/haemoglobin and platelet count. The shadowing seen in this case was due to *Pneumocystis carinii* pneumonia. This was confirmed with bronchial washings obtained at bronchoscopy. Often there is simultaneous infection with another pathogen. *Pneumocystis carinii* pneumonia affects immunosuppressed patients, including those with AIDS with a CD4 count below $0.2 \times 10^9/l$. Treatment is with pentamidine or co-trimoxazole.

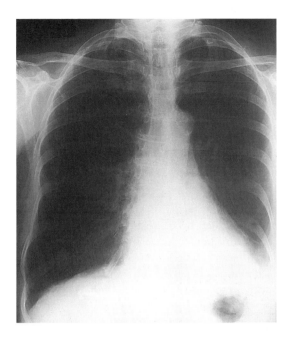

Questions

This 81-year-old woman was referred to the out patient clinic with a history of recent worsening of dyspnoea and a cough with haemoptysis.

a. What does her chest radiograph show?
b. How would you investigate her further?
c. Why was she also under surgical follow-up?

Answers

a. The left hilum is displaced inferiorly and the heart deviated to the left. There is a triangular opacity behind the heart. These findings all indicate left lower lobe collapse. There is also the impression of a mass at the lower pole of the hilum. The right breast shadow is absent due to a previous mastectomy for breast carcinoma.

b. Bronchoscopy and computed tomography (CT) scan of her chest.

c. She was under surgical follow-up for the breast carcinoma.

Discussion

The hilar mass causing left lower lobe collapse in this case could represent a metastasis from her previous breast carcinoma (endobronchial metastases from breast primaries are well recognized) or she may have a primary lung carcinoma. Bronchoscopy with transbronchial biopsy and washings would help to make a histological diagnosis. Clinical signs of left lower lobe collapse include deviation of the trachea to the left, reduced expansion on the left with dullness at the left base and decreased air entry. She may also have supraclavicular or axillary lymph nodes due to metastatic disease.

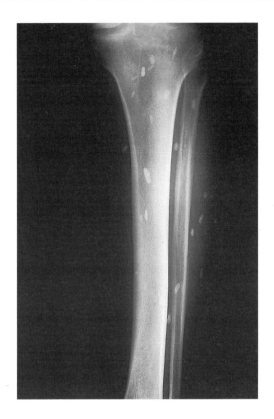

Questions

This is a radiograph of a 74-year-old Second World War veteran.

a. What is the cause of this appearance?
b. In which theatre of war did he serve?

Answers

a. There are oval calcific opacities, many with a central lucency, in the soft tissues. These are aligned with their long axis in the line of the muscle fibres. The appearance is typical of cysticercosis.

b. One of the endemic areas is South East Asia.

Discussion

The calcification is in the dead cysts of *Taenia solium*, the pork tapeworm. The adult lives in the human gut. Eggs are shed in the faeces and the larvae develop in the pig (intermediate host). Sometimes humans can become infested with the larvae (cysticerci) through cross infection from people harbouring the adult worm, or through contaminated food or water. The cysticerci are found in the muscle, and in organs such as the brain, eyes and heart. The main effects are neurological, especially epilepsy. Endemic areas include South East Asia, India, Central and South America and South Africa.

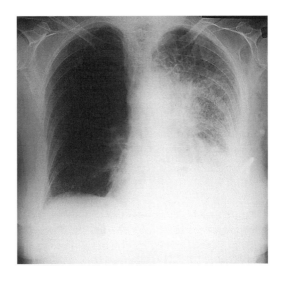

Questions

This 71-year-old lady presents with increasing shortness of breath.

a. List two abnormalities on her chest X-ray
b. What is the most likely underlying aetiology?

Answers

a. There is a mass at the left hilum with some loss of volume of that lung and extensive linear shadowing which radiates from the hilum. The hilar mass is a primary bronchial carcinoma, although lymphadeno-pathy could give a similar appearance. The pulmonary shadowing is lymphangitis carcinomatosa.

b. The commonest tumours which cause lymphangitis are lung and breast carcinomas.

Discussion

The cause of lymphangitis carcinomatosa is tumour infiltration of the lymphatics which produces the linear shadowing observed on the chest X-ray. It is usually unilateral but can be bilateral. Pulmonary oedema can produce similar shadowing, but this is usually bilateral and it would not account for the hilar mass. The patient presents classically with dyspnoea which is difficult to treat. On examination there is reduced expansion of the lungs and crackles or wheezes can be heard. It is important to exclude any evidence of left ventricular failure or infection which can be treated. Bronchodilators can be given if there is an obstructive element to the respiratory distress. Radiotherapy may be helpful depending upon the underlying aetiology. Treatment is usually symptomatic, however, and the prognosis is poor. Lymphangitis has a characteristic appearance on high resolution CT of the lungs. There is predominantly smooth thicken-ing of the interlobular septa and centrilobular structures with some nodularity. CT would also show the hilar mass and any lymphadenopathy in more detail.

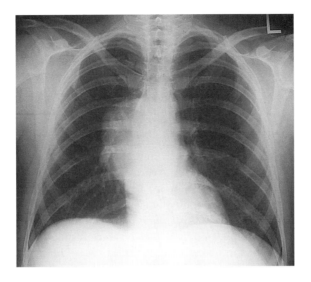

Question

This 26-year-old man had this chest radiograph to confirm resolution of a chest infection.

What is the incidental finding?

Answer

Bronchogenic cyst.

Discussion

There is a large right sided mediastinal mass present. The right heart border and ascending aorta are still clearly seen so it must lie behind these. The hilar vessels are not all seen, however, so it must contact the hilum and extend posteriorly. It is smooth, non lobulated and contains no calcification. No splaying of the ribs is seen (which, if present, would have favoured a neurogenic tumour lying posteriorly). This is a bronchogenic cyst. It a is developmental cystic duplication of the bronchial tree. Most are in the carina/hilar region and lie posterior to the trachea on a lateral radiograph. In infants they produce respiratory distress due to compression of the major airways, but in older children and adults they are usually asymptomatic. On CT a thin walled cystic structure is the usual finding. The differential diagnosis in this case would include a neurenteric cyst. This is another type of duplication cyst related to the oesophagus and sometimes associated with congenital vertebral anomalies. Other possible diagnoses include: lymphadenopathy (though one may expect a lymph node mass to be lobulated), a central lung carcinoma (less likely in so young a patient), or a hydatid cyst (the main cyst may contain daughter cysts) – visible on CT. Immunodiagnostic tests may show antibodies to *Echinococcus granulosus*.

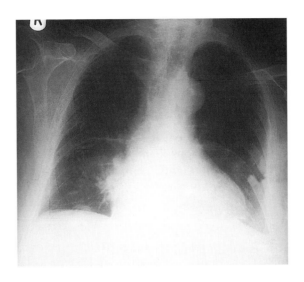

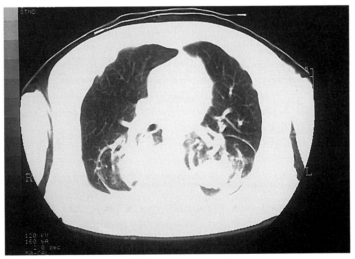

Questions

a. What abnormalities are present on the chest radiograph of this 77-year-old former shipyard worker (list two)?

b. What does the CT scan demonstrate?

Answers

a. There are pleural plaques visible (e.g. on the right hemidiaphragm and in the right mid zone). These are due to previous asbestos exposure during his years as a shipyard worker. This patient has apparent masses at both lung bases (that on the left is behind the cardiac shadow). The obvious worry here is the possibility of lung cancer.

b. This shows two areas of folded lung (also known as round atelectasis). The appearance of the fibrosis and vessels curving into the mass is typical. This is a benign condition not infrequently found in patients who have been exposed to asbestos.

Discussion

Exposure to asbestos can produce pulmonary fibrosis (asbestosis), lung cancer and pleural mesothelioma. Pleural plaques and pleural thickening on a chest X-ray indicates that a patient has been exposed to asbestos but the patient may be asymptomatic. Similarly a patient's sputum may contain asbestos bodies which can be seen at microscopy and these are merely an indication that the patient has previously been exposed to asbestos and not that they have necessarily developed any of the complications of exposure. It is important therefore in respiratory diseases to take an occupational history and also, if the patient is a woman, the occupation of her husband is important as wives are exposed to asbestos by laundering their husband's clothes.

Clinical features of asbestosis include: dyspnoea, cough, sputum and attacks of bronchitis. Pulmonary function tests may show an obstructive defect in the early stages. If pulmonary fibrosis develops the classical signs of pulmonary fibrosis (finger clubbing, fine basal late inspiratory crackles, decreased lung expansion, type I respiratory failure and a restrictive pulmonary defect) should be sought. Patients may also develop cor pulmonale in association with the chronic respiratory disease.

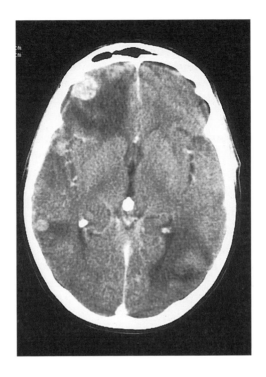

Questions

This 62-year-old woman presented with increasing confusion. She had had an operation 2 years previously which was complicated by swelling in her left arm and hand. She had complained of backache and weight loss for 6 months.

a. What is this investigation?
b. What does it show?
c. What is the possible cause of her backache?
d. What operation did she have 2 years ago?

Answers

a. An enhanced CT scan of brain.
   It is important to mention that it is an enhanced scan – i.e. contrast has been given intravenously. This should be indicated on scans by the +C; in some units the name of the contrast medium is printed on the scan.

b. There are four areas of abnormal enhancement present, three in the right cerebral hemisphere and one in the left. These appear as white, round or irregular masses with surrounding low attenuation (dark grey) which is cerebral oedema. These lesions are cerebral metastases.

c. Bony secondaries.

d. The operation she had 2 years previously was a left mastectomy for breast carcinoma with axillary node clearance. This has resulted in lymphoedema of the left arm which is a common complication of a radical mastectomy. It is often difficult to treat and causes considerable discomfort to the patient.

Discussion

The fact that there are multiple lesions on the CT scan and the previous history makes it likely that these lesions are metastatic deposits from a primary carcinoma of breast. The other common tumour which metastasizes to brain is lung. Primary brain tumours are usually (but not always) solitary.

The clinical presentation of cerebral metastases depends upon their site. There may be symptoms due to raised intracranial pressure, e.g. morning headache, nausea, vomiting, confusion, apathy, drowsiness. Epilepsy occurs in 30% of cases, particularly when the frontal or temporal lobes are involved. Focal neurological signs depend upon the site of the lesions. A sixth nerve palsy is a sign of raised intracranial pressure and is a 'false localizing sign'. Symptoms may also occur due to associated hyponatraemia due to inappropriate ADH secretion which is associated with cerebral lesions. Hyponatraemia causes malaise, apathy, confusion, drowsiness and ultimately seizures.

This patient clearly has metastatic disease and the outlook is poor.

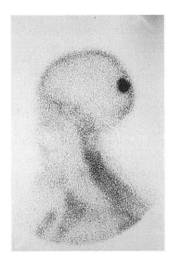 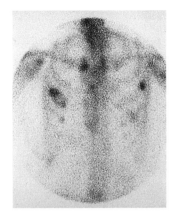

Questions

This 70-year-old woman complained of recurrent nose bleeds and chest infections. On examination she was cachectic and had several bruises on her legs. Her blood results were as follows:

- Haemoglobin 9.1 g/dl
- White cell count $2.0 \times 10^9/l$
- Platelets $30 \times 10^9/l$
- Sodium 140 mmol/l
- Potassium 4.5 mmol/l
- Urea 8.9 mmol/l
- Calcium 2.9 mmol/l
- Albumin 30 g/l
- ALP 400 IU/l
- AST 800 IU/l
- Bilirubin 80 μmol/l
- INR 2.0.

a. What is this investigation?
b. What are the abnormalities and what is the cause?
c. Explain her blood results.

Answers

a. An isotope bone scan.

b. There are multiple areas of increased uptake due to bony metastases.

c. There is a pancytopenia due to bone marrow involvement by tumour. The abnormal liver function tests are probably due to liver metastases. Corrected calcium is high (3.0 mmol/l) and this and the raised ALP are due to bony secondaries. The INR is increased due to impaired liver function and this and the thrombocytopenia will give rise to her bleeding diathesis.

Discussion

In nuclear medicine imaging a radioisotope (in this case ^{99m}Tc) is linked to a carrier molecule that is taken up by the structure to be imaged. In the case of bone, methylene diphosphonate (MDP) is used. This is taken up in normal bone but areas of abnormally high bone turnover show increased uptake. This patient has several such areas (in the skull vault, cervical spine and ribs). There are many causes of increased uptake (e.g. fractures, Paget's disease, tumour, osteomyelitis, arthritides) but the pattern here indicates bony metastases. She had a known breast carcinoma.

The static phase of a bone scan is carried out 3 hours after injection of the isotope. 50–60% of the dose is taken up by bone and the rest renally excreted. To improve bone to soft tissue contrast, and to reduce the radiation dose to the bladder, the patient is asked to drink a large amount of liquid and to empty the bladder prior to the scan.

A radioisotope bone scan is more sensitive to pathology than plain radiographs which only show visible changes when there has been a 50% increase or decrease in bone calcium. The bone scan is less specific, however, and interpretation must be in the light of the clinical history and the appearance of plain radiographs of any abnormal areas.

Because MDP is renally excreted there is increased soft tissue uptake in renal failure which reduces contrast on the scan. Normally the kidneys are visible on bone scan images but another situation where they are not is when there is very high bone uptake. This is termed a super scan and can be seen with bony metastases from carcinoma of the prostate. As the increased uptake is so widespread it can be overlooked. The absent renal uptake gives a clue, as does the reduced time to acquire the necessary count level for the scan. Sometimes the skull can also seem to be absent due to greatly increased uptake elsewhere in the skeleton dominating the received counts. Another trap is the area of reduced uptake due to destructive bony lesion (such as myeloma, but also in some carcinomas). This is harder to see than an area of increased uptake.

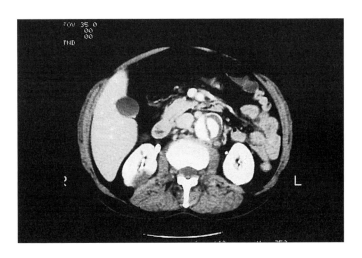

Questions

This is a single slice from a CT scan of the chest and abdomen performed on a 62-year-old man with severe chest and interscapular pain. His chest radiograph was abnormal.

a. What does the CT scan show?
b. What is the diagnosis?
c. What are the typical chest X-ray signs of this condition?

Answers

a. There is slight dilatation of the abdominal aorta with an intimal flap dividing the false and two lumens.

b. This is the appearance of an aortic dissection.

c. Signs of this that may have been seen on the chest radiograph are enlargement of the aortic knuckle and an apical cap of soft tissue density on the left (at the lung apex). If the aortic wall is calcified, then the outer edge of the aortic knuckle may be seen to extend significantly more laterally than the rim of calcification which is another clue.

Discussion

Dissection of the aorta is classified according to its point of origin and extent. The DeBakey classification is as follows:

- **Type 1.** Begins in the ascending aorta and extends distally beyond the ligamentum arteriosum
- **Type 2.** Begins in the ascending aorta but stops proximal to the brachiocephalic trunk
- **Type 3.** Begins at or distal to the ligamentum arteriosum and extends distally (or occasionally proximally to the aortic arch).

A variation on this classification is:

- **Type A.** DeBakey types 1 and 2, and type 3 if it propagates retrogradely
- **Type B.** DeBakey types 3 dissections which only propagate distally.

This latter classification system was based on therapy, with type A being treated surgically and type B medically. As a result this simplified system is more useful.

Dissecting aortic aneurysms are more common in patients with atherosclerosis, hypertension and disorders of connective tissue (e.g. Marfan's syndrome). The patient complains of severe central chest pain and interscapular pain. Pulses in the arms may be absent or asymmetrical depending upon the stage of the dissection and blood pressure should be measured in each arm. It is important to make an early diagnosis and CT scanning or transoesophageal echocardiography is the investigation of choice. The patient should be closely monitored and, if hypertensive, the blood pressure should be carefully controlled. A cardiothoracic surgeon should be involved in the management at diagnosis as surgical intervention is often required.

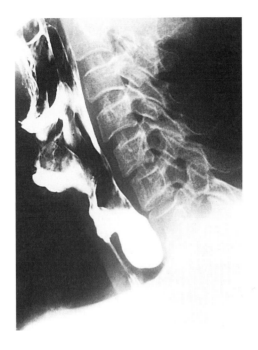

Questions

This is one film from a barium swallow series performed on a 65-year-old woman with dysphagia which she localized to her throat.

a. What does the film show?

b. List two other symptoms she may have.

Answers

a. A pharyngeal pouch (Zenker's diverticulum).

b. Regurgitation, symptoms due to aspiration pneumonia which is recurrent and common.

Discussion

A pharyngeal pouch (Zenker's diverticulum) is a common cause of high dysphagia. Food which collects in the pouch may later regurgitate and cause a foul taste or aspiration or choking. It may also become large enough to be palpable, usually on the left side of the neck. The diverticulum arises through a weakness (Killian's dehiscence) between the oblique and transverse fibres of the inferior constrictor muscle of the pharynx. Impaired relaxation of this muscle (cricopharyngeus) causes the pulsion diverticulum to form. This then passes posteriorly and inferiorly (sometimes even into the mediastinum). This impaired relaxation of cricopharyngeus can cause dysphagia even without a diverticulum. It is also detectable on barium swallow examination, as are some other causes of cervical dysphagia such as a post-cricoid web, pharyngocoele, carcinoma and lower oesophageal problems which sometimes present as if they were higher than they in fact are. A pharyngeal pouch is more common in men and usually occurs in the elderly. Treatment is excision of the pouch combined with a myotomy of the cricopharyngeus muscle.

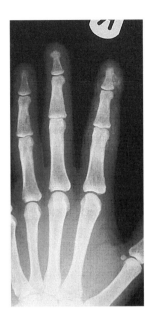

Questions

This patient complained of polyuria and polydipsia for 3 months and was admitted to hospital with acute colicky abdominal pain.

a. Name two abnormalities on the X-ray.
b. What is the diagnosis?
c. What is the cause of her symptoms?

Answers

a. There is soft tissue calcification (seen here in just the index finger) and erosions of the tufts of the distal phalanges.

b. Hyperparathyroidism.

c. Hypercalcaemia causes polyuria and polydipsia; this results in dehydration and constipation can occur which could be the cause of this patient's abdominal pain. However, the most likely reason for her 'colicky' abdominal pain is renal colic due to renal stones which are secondary to the hypercalcaemia.

Discussion

Erosion of the tufts of the distal phalanges is seen in a number of conditions including hyperparathyroidism, scleroderma, psoriatic arthropathy, Raynaud's disease, various causes of neuropathy (including diabetes mellitus and syringomyelia), epidermolysis bullosa, porphyria, trauma and thermal injuries. Of these hyperparathyroidism and scleroderma also cause soft tissue calcification (as can trauma). Soft tissue calcification is commoner in secondary than in primary hyperparathyroidism. Classically, in hyperparathyroidism, as well as soft tissue calcification and erosion of the distal phalanages there are subperiosteal erosions occurring usually on the radial side of the middle phalanx. There may be lucent areas in bone, cysts also known as brown tumours or osteitis fibrosa cystica, loss of the lamina dura of the teeth, pepper pot skull or generalized osteopenia.

Primary hyperparathyroidism is most commonly the result of a parathyroid gland adenoma (90%). Excess parathyroid hormone increases plasma calcium levels by increasing calcium absorption from the gut, increasing mobilization of calcium from bone and reducing renal calcium excretion. A parathyroid adenoma may also be part of a multiple endocrine adenomatosis syndrome and can be associated with benign adenomas of the pancreatic islets, pituitary tumours, thyroid and adrenal cortical tumours. It may also be associated with a pheochromocytoma and a calcitonin producing medullary carcinoma of the thyroid gland.

In primary hyperparathyroidism the calcium is raised and phosphate level reduced. Treatment depends upon symptoms and the calcium level. It is usual to consider a parathyroidectomy when the calcium level is above 3 mmol/l and there are symptoms.

Secondary hyperparathyroidism is part of the spectrum of renal osteodystrophy, as is osteomalacia/rickets. In this case there is hypocalcaemia and hypophosphataemia (unlike primary or tertiary hyperparathyroidism where serum calcium is raised).

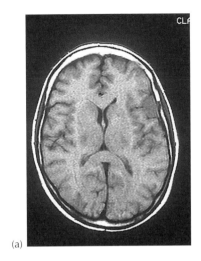
(a)

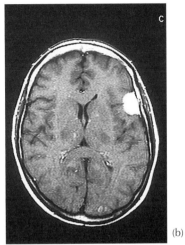
(b)

Question

These are two images from an MRI scan of the brain of a 45-year-old woman. They are both T1-weighted. Section (a) is unenhanced and section (b) is at the same level following intravenous gadolinium.

What abnormality is shown?

Answer

The patient has a meningioma which shows atypical appearance, being iso-intense with the brain on the unenhanced image and enhancing strongly after intravenous gadolinium. This enhancement is homogenous and there is evidence of extension along the dura. The absence of associated oedema fits well with a benign slow growing lesion (although they can also have oedema around them in some cases).

Discussion

MRI shows intracranial tumours better than CT. However, it may miss intratumoural calcification unless this is very extensive. Meningiomas represent about 15% of intracranial tumours (being less common than gliomas or metastases). They are commoner in women and benign in nature, though malignant change can occur. They may erode underlying bone or cause a hyperostotic reaction. Their vascular supply may be visible on imaging. Common sites are over the cerebral convexity (especially adjacent to the falx and superior sagittal sinus) and at the skull base (especially sphenoid ridge and parasella region). Less commonly they may be intraventricular, along the sheath of one of the cranial nerves (especially the optic nerve), or in the spinal canal. Clinically the patient may present with many symptoms mainly depending upon the location of the tumour. However, there may be symptoms due to raised intracranial pressure (early morning headache, nausea, confusion, drowsiness, sixth cranial nerve palsy). The presentation may be with a fit which occurs in about 30% of cases, particularly when the frontal and temporal lobes are involved. They can also be asymptomatic. Meningiomas may be surgically resected but they can recur. Radiotherapy or just observation with follow-up scans are other possible lines of management, depending on the case.

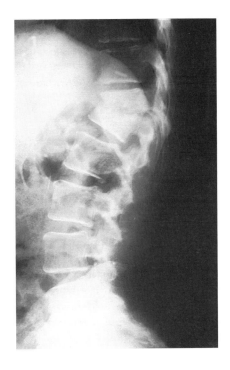

Question

This 46-year-old man had had backache for several months; it was becoming progressively worse. On examination there was tenderness in the thoracolumbar junction. Blood test results were as follows: ESR 96 mm/hr, Hb 13.6 g/dl, white cell count 14.0×10^9/l.

What is the diagnosis?

Answer

The lateral plain radiograph of the spine shows loss of disc space and destruction of the end plates of the adjacent vertebral bodies at the T12/L1 level. The appearances are those of discitis.

Discussion

Discitis may result from spread of infection from elsewhere by septic emboli or it may be post surgical. As with osteomyelitis elsewhere, radiological changes are slow to develop and may delay diagnosis for several weeks. Radioisotope bone scans and MRI are more sensitive. The infection may be pyogenic (especially *Staphylococcus aureus*) or tuberculous. Successful treatment of a pyogenic infection with antibiotics may result in worsening of the radiological appearance, despite clinical improvement, due to replacement of devitalized bone by granulation tissue and reduction in inflammation revealing the extent of disc destruction and causing a further loss of height. Later new bone formation may fuse the vertebral bodies. Unless a paravertebral/psoas abscess has developed, fever, constitutional symptoms and a raised white count are not features of spinal infection. Their absence should not discourage one from making the diagnosis. Disruption of bone can lead to cord compression which should be guarded against. It is often necessary to use a spinal brace to ensure stability of the spine. The legs should be examined neurologically daily to ensure that the spinal cord has not become involved as surgical intervention may then be required.

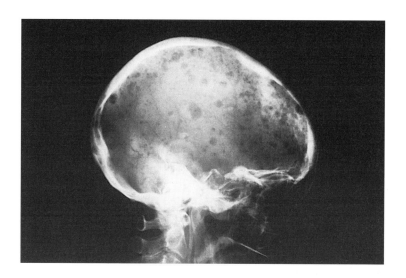

Questions

This is the skull radiograph of a 65-year-old woman who complained of tiredness and weight loss. Investigations were as follows:

- Haemoglobin 10.1 g/dl
- White cell count $3.6 \times 10^9/l$
- MCV 88 fl
- ESR 70 mm/hr
- ALP 400 IU/l
- AST 20 IU/l
- Urine Bence Jones protein negative.

a. What is the abnormality and what is the most likely cause?
b. Give two possible reasons for her anaemia.

Answers

a. There are multiple lytic lesions in the skull vault due to metastases. The tumours which are most commonly responsible for lytic bony metastases are breast and bronchus.

b. She has a normocytic anaemia. This may be due to chronic disease or infiltration of the bone marrow by the tumour causing bone marrow suppression and this may be the reason for the slightly reduced white cell count.

Discussion

Metastases may be lytic, sclerotic, or mixed density on plain radiographs. If a single lesion is found, a radioisotope bone scan may help by showing others elsewhere in the skeleton. Metastases usually show increased uptake of the isotope, but myeloma can be harder to see as there is often decreased uptake. Multiple myeloma is due to infiltration of the bone marrow by plasma cell malignancy. Laboratory tests can show anaemia, raised ESR, elevation of one class of immunoglobulin, or heavy or light chains in the serum (with suppression of other immunoglobulin classes), or light chains in the urine. Also there may be raised serum urea, creatinine, calcium and uric acid levels. However, alkaline phosphatase levels are usually normal, so the raised level in this case is further support for the diagnosis of metastases.

Bony secondaries usually present with pain which also may be due to a pathological fracture. Bony destruction from metastases results in hypercalcaemia and its symptoms (polyuria, polydypsia, renal stones, constipation, depression). Bone pain from metastases often responds to treatment with non-steroidal anti-inflammatory drugs and, if necessary, palliative radiotherapy can be helpful. Pathological fractures require internal fixation.

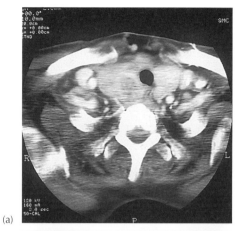

(a)

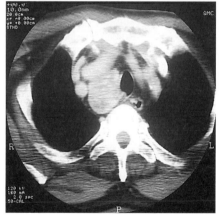

(b)

Questions

This 45-year-old lady complains of difficulty with breathing and on examination she is found to have stridor.

a. What do these CT scans show?
b. List one other symptom she may have.

Answers

a. There is enlargement of the thyroid gland which surrounds and narrows the trachea (Fig. a) and retrosternal extension of the goitre (Fig. b).

b. Dysphagia (due to oesophageal compression). Breathlessness, however, is a more common symptom.

Discussion

In addition to standard blood tests of thyroid function, the imaging investigation of thyroid enlargement starts with an ultrasound scan and a radioisotope study. Ultrasound shows the anatomy of the gland and confirms enlargement. It will show if the thyroid texture is homogeneous (normal) or multinodular, and tell solid lumps from cysts. A cyst could then be drained. A nuclear medicine scan using ^{99m}Tc pertechnetate demonstrates the function of the gland as it is taken up by functioning thyroid tissue. It should be reported along with the ultrasound scan, as a 'cold' area (with no uptake) is expected if it corresponds to a cyst, but if associated with a solitary solid nodule is worrying with respect to malignancy. However, some adenomas are also non-functioning. Biopsy is required in the case of solid, non-functioning thyroid nodules. CT is usually not needed but can be useful to assess retrosternal extension and tracheal compression, as here. Preoperative assessment should include laryngoscopy to assess the vocal cords and extent of laryngeal compression.

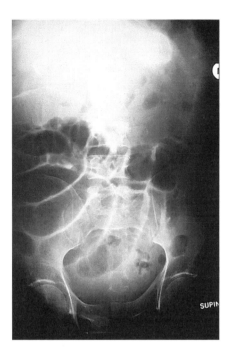

Questions

This man had suffered from dyspepsia for a few years prior to presenting as an emergency with more severe upper abdominal pain.

a. What is the abnormality on the abdominal X-ray?
b. What is the most likely cause?

Answers

a. There are dilated loops of small bowel with both sides of the bowel wall visible. This is a sign of free peritoneal air on a supine radiograph.

b. Perforated duodenal ulcer.

Discussion

This supine abdominal film demonstrates free gas in the peritoneal space due to a ruptured viscus. Gas under the diaphragm would be apparent on the erect chest X-ray. The commonest cause of gas in the peritoneum is postoperative but in this case the patient had complained of abdominal pain. The most likely cause of sudden onset of abdominal pain is a perforated duodenal ulcer, especially given the history of dyspepsia. Diverticula in the colon can also produce a similar picture but this is less common. Perforation is a complication of a duodenal ulcer rather than a gastric ulcer. The other main complications of duodenal ulcers are bleeding and pyloric stenosis. There are certain clinical features which can distinguish between duodenal and gastric ulcers. Duodenal ulceration usually produces a history of periodic epigastric pain which awakens the patient at 3 a.m. and is relieved by food, milk and antacids. The patients suffer several weeks of pain with periods of remission. As the pain is relieved by food, the patients tend to gain weight. Gastric ulcer pain is also epigastric but is antagonized by food and is often associated with anorexia, vomiting and weight loss. Gastric ulcers can be malignant and endoscopy and biopsy is essential. A further endoscopy after 2 months to ensure healing is also necessary. In this case, where there is perforation, urgent laparotomy and oversewing of the duodenal ulcer is required. Vagotomy is usually also performed. Long term H_2 antagonists to prevent recurrence are indicated.

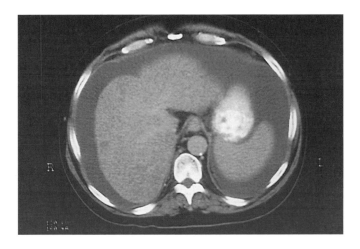

Questions

This is a CT scan of a 56-year-old publican. He complained of upper abdominal pain.

a. Name two abnormalities on the CT scan.
b. What is the diagnosis?
c. List two possible causes of his abdominal pain.
d. List three clinical signs he may have.

Answers

a. There is evidence of ascites (fluid is the black area on the scan surrounding the abdominal organs). The liver is abnormal in texture and irregular which is the appearance of cirrhosis.

b. Hepatic cirrhosis causing portal hypertension and ascites. Alcoholism is the commonest cause of hepatic cirrhosis in the UK and is the case here.

c. He may have abdominal pain due to distension from the ascites or he may have an associated peptic ulcer which is common in alcoholics.

d. Signs of ascites include abdominal distension, shifting dullness and a fluid thrill. He may also have clinical signs of chronic liver disease: finger clubbing, leukonychia, Dupuytren's contracture, palmar erythema, jaundice, spider naevi, hypopigmentation, gynaecomastia, loss of body hair, testicular atrophy, purpura.

Discussion

This is an image from a CT scan of the upper abdomen. It shows the presence of ascites. The liver is abnormal, inhomogeneous in texture with a slightly knobbly border. The patient has cirrhosis of the liver due to alcoholism. CT may also show splenomegaly and venous collaterals. All these features can be seen on ultrasound which also allows assessment of the portal vein using Doppler examination to show any flow reversal. As there is an increased risk of hepatocellular carcinoma one also needs to look out for evidence of this on either CT or ultrasound. Although this CT scan appearance is typical of hepatic cirrhosis this diagnosis is a pathological one and implies a liver biopsy has been performed. The cirrhosis associated with alcoholism is usually micronodular in type. There are many causes of cirrhosis as follows:

- Infection (hepatitis B, C, etc.)
- Toxic chemicals (alcohol, drugs e.g. methyldopa)
- Immunological (primary biliary cirrhosis, chronic active hepatitis)
- Prolonged cholestasis
- Metabolic (haemochromatosis, hepatolenticular degeneration, galactosaemia, glycogen storage diseases, tyrosinosis, α_1-antitrypsin deficiency)
- Venous congestion (cardiac failure, hepatic vein obstruction)
- Idiopathic

● Miscellaneous (hereditary haemorrhagic telangectasia, sickle cell disease, jejunoileal bypass).

Cirrhosis is the commonest cause of portal hypertension and when this develops there is usually some evidence of hepatocellular failure. Portal hypertension results in the production of varices at the portal systemic anastomoses (e.g. oesophageal varices, haemorrhoids, caput medusae). Bleeding oesophageal varices carry a mortality of 50% despite treatment.

Ascites occurs when cirrhosis becomes decompensated. Patients with ascites tend to have a low urine sodium level. Other biochemical findings in cirrhosis include hypoalbuminaemia and raised serum levels of γ-glutamyl transaminase, aspartate transaminase and bilirubin.

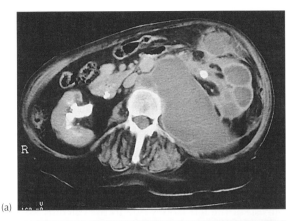

(a)

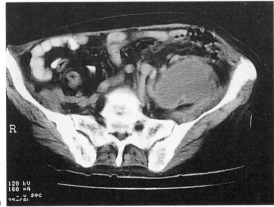

(b)

Questions

This 76-year-old man presented with abdominal pain and vomiting. On examination there was left-sided tenderness and fullness and he was unable to straighten the left hip. He was pyrexial, had a raised white count and mild anaemia.

a. List three abnormalities on the CT scan.
b. What is the treatment?

Answers

a. The left kidney is hydronephrotic with marked cortical loss indicating a long standing problem. There is no excretion of contrast and a calculus is seen (Fig. a). The psoas muscle is markedly swollen and of low attenuation. This can be followed down into the pelvis (Fig. b). This patient has a psoas abscess secondary to pyelonephritis.

b. The management includes blood cultures and an MSSU as the patient is clearly septic and microbiological evidence should be gathered. The patient should then receive intravenous broad spectrum antibiotics. The psoas abscess should be drained and this can be performed under ultrasound or CT scan control. Recurrent infection has occurred with hydronephrosis of the left kidney due to the calculus which can also be seen. Lithotripsy could be considered to remove this to prevent further infection. A nephrostomy may also be required to drain the left hydronephrosis. However, in this case the non-functioning kidney is unlikely to recover significantly and nephrectomy may be the best option.

Discussion

A psoas abscess can result from pyelonephritis or a spinal or paraspinal infection. The psoas muscle flexes the hip joint and therefore the hip is usually in fixed flexion and the patient experiences pain on extension of the hip. If a hydronephrosis is present the kidney is usually palpable and tender. The pyelonephritis produces symptoms of dysuria, frequency and loin pain. The patient often has rigors and vomiting. The commonest organism (80% of cases) is *Escherichia coli* but all other organisms (proteus, staphylococcus, pseudomonas, klebsiella) can be involved and these are usually associated with structural abnormalities. Precipitating causes for infection, as well as structural abnormality, include pregnancy and diabetes mellitus. An episode of pyelonephritis should be fully investigated to prevent further episodes which could result in renal damage and its complications (e.g. hypertension).

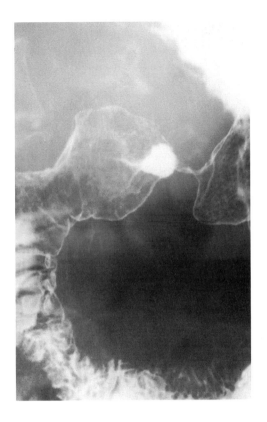

Questions

This 38-year-old man presented with a long standing history of epigastric pain.

a. What does the barium meal show?
b. What treatment should he receive?

Answers

a. This film from the barium meal series shows the first and second parts of the duodenum. There is an ulcer crater in the duodenal cap with surrounding oedema and radiating folds.

b. He should receive general advice on healthy living, e.g. reduce alcohol intake, stop smoking, reduce weight, healthy diet. He should also receive a 6-week course of H_2 antagonists (e.g. ranitidine). If there is evidence of *Helicobacter pylori* infection then this is associated with recurrent duodenal ulceration and eradication therapy with antibiotics should also be given. However, there is no indication that infection has been sought in this case and it is usually found at endoscopy and biopsy when the organisms are seen on histology. There are other investigations (e.g. breath testing to detect *H. pylori* infection) but these are often expensive.

Discussion

The cap is the commonest site for a duodenal ulcer, though they can occur in the immediate post-bulbar region and the second part of the duodenum. Scarring from the recurrent ulceration or deformity due to previous surgery can mask an active ulcer crater and a barium meal is less reliable in assessing such cases, especially anastomotic ulcers at the site of a gastroenterostomy. Fewer barium meal examinations are now performed as they are being replaced with endoscopy. However, a barium meal can be more helpful to assess some complications of ulcers (e.g. pyloric stenosis).

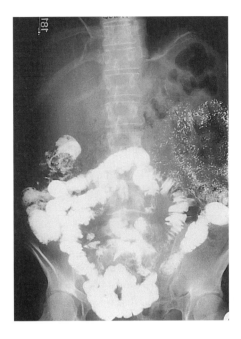

Questions

This 61-year-old lady presented with diarrhoea and weight loss. She had a palpable mass in the lower abdomen. She had been on a special diet since the age of 10 years when her initial presentation was failure to grow (short stature). Her full blood count revealed: haemoglobin 8.7 g/dl, red cell count = 3.09×10^{12}/l, white cell count = 3.8×10^{9}/l. This is a film from her small bowel series.

a. What does the film show?
b. What is the most likely diagnosis?
c. What is the special diet she is on and what is this for?

Answers

a. There are several adjacent loops of ileum which are grossly abnormal. The bowel loops are pushed apart by a mass and the involved loops are markedly irregular and distorted.

b. Small bowel lymphoma.

c. Gluten free diet. Coeliac disease.

Discussion

The main differential is between Crohn's disease and lymphoma. Other possibilities are carcinoid tumour or metastases (especially from carcinoma of the ovary, gastrointestinal tract, breast and melanoma). Bowel involvement in lymphomas is usually in non-Hodgkin's lymphoma. It occurs by direct extension from mesenteric nodes, or primary bowel lymphoma. The latter is more common and is a complication of coeliac disease. Patients with coeliac disease also have a higher incidence of carcinoma of the bowel. Coeliac disease is due to a sensitivity to wheat gluten, barley and rye. There is an increased incidence in relatives and is associated with HLA B8 and DRW3. Antibodies to reticulin are often present and there is an association with dermatitis herpetiformis. Clinically the presentation is in childhood or late adult life and the symptoms and signs are due to malabsorption: steatorrhoea, weight loss, abdominal distension and pain, and vitamin deficiency. On examination the patient looks cachectic and often has pigmented scaly skin with a distended abdomen and increased bowel sounds. Finger clubbing may be present and there may be specific signs of vitamin deficiencies (e.g. subacute combined degeneration of the cord due to B_{12} deficiency). The diagnosis is made by duodenal biopsy which classically shows sub-total villous atrophy. Treatment is with a lifelong gluten free diet.

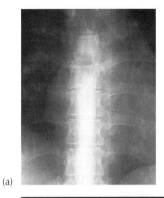

(a)

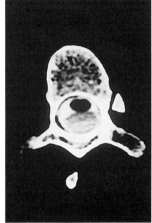

(b)

Questions

This 52-year-old woman presented with a progressive spastic paraplegia. She had first noticed some weakness about a year prior to this examination. On examination there was weakness in both lower limbs and a sensory level at T8.

a. What examinations are shown in Figures a and b?
b. What abnormality is demonstrated?
c. What is the differential diagnosis?
d. What alternative examination would be used more often now?

Answers

a. Figure a is from a myelogram and b is a CT scan performed with the myelographic contrast present.

b. They show an intradural, extra medullary mass seen as a filling defect.

c. The two most common tumours in this location are neurofibroma and meningioma. Neurofibromata more commonly cause bony erosion. In this case the tumour is a meningioma. They are commoner in women and spinal meningiomas are most often thoracic in location as here.

d. Myelography has now been largely replaced by magnetic resonance imaging (MRI) but is still performed when MRI is contraindicated by severe claustrophobia, the presence of a cardiac pacemaker, some cardiac valve replacements, cochlear implants, intracranial vascular clips, intraocular metallic foreign body, etc.

Discussion

Spastic paraparesis is a neurosurgical emergency and if left untreated will result in permanent neurological damage. Treatment within 2 days of the onset of symptoms may avoid permanent damage to the spinal cord. In this case neurosurgical decompression is required. If there is surrounding inflammation dexamethasone should also be prescribed to reduce the pressure on the spinal cord. In the case of inoperable malignant spinal tumours which may be metastatic radiotherapy may alleviate symptoms.

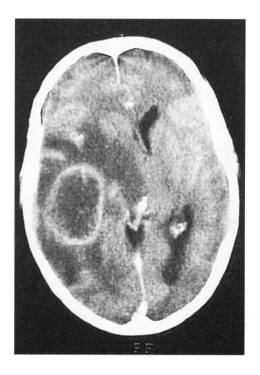

Questions

This 62-year-old man presented with a history of adult onset epilepsy and, more recently, headaches, vomiting and left-sided weakness. The onset of these was gradual rather than sudden.

a. What does this image from a contrast enhanced CT scan of the brain show?
b. What is the most likely diagnosis?

Answers

a. There is a ring enhancing mass in the right parietal lobe. This has a cystic centre and considerable surrounding oedema. There is mass effect with compression of the right lateral ventricle and midline shift to the left.

b. This appearance could be due to a cerebral abscess or a tumour. The most likely diagnosis is that of cystic glioma. Gliomas are very infiltrative tumours and the area of enhancement does not mark the edge of the tumour. The oedematous area will be extensively infiltrated.

Discussion

Gliomas are the commonest primary brain tumours. There are several histological types; most are glioblastoma multiforme or astrocytomas. There are two peak ages of incidence: childhood (5–10 years) and adulthood (50–60 years). The incidence overall is 5–15/100 000 per year. The majority (90%) occur in the frontal, parietal or temporal lobes. The symptoms and signs they produce depend upon their location. There are often symptoms and signs due to raised intracranial pressure.

Surgery is not always appropriate for gliomas as the operative risks may outweigh the benefits. The main purposes of surgery are: to establish histological diagnosis, remove tumour to relieve raised intracranial pressure and neurological damage, and cure. The last is uncommon. Adjuvant radiotherapy with surgery can be effective in treating residual tumour and improve survival. Gliomas respond to chemotherapy. The patient is therefore usually informed jointly by the neurosurgeon, radiotherapist and oncologist so that the best treatment option is decided for each individual case.

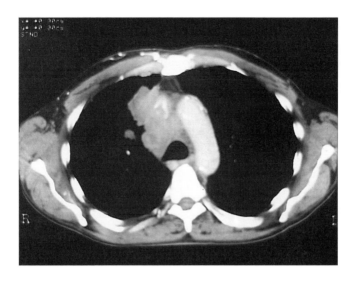

Questions

This 65-year-old man is a lifelong smoker who presents with a history of shortness of breath and weight loss.

a. What does this contrast enhanced CT scan show?
b. What is the diagnosis?

Answers

a. There is a lobulated mass in the mediastinum at the level of the aortic arch. The superior vena cava is compressed to a narrow slit and dilated veins are seen over the chest wall. The lobulated mass represents lymphadenopathy. It is causing superior vena caval obstruction which is almost always, as here, due to malignancy.

b. Bronchial carcinoma (metastatic).

Discussion

Superior vena caval compression is usually caused by enlarged lymph nodes most commonly due to metastatic bronchial carcinoma. It can be due to lymphoma or other metastatic tumours or rarely a fibrous band in the mediastinum. The patient usually develops swelling of the face, neck and upper limbs with dilated veins on the neck and chest due to obstruction in venous return. Headache, breathlessness and dizziness are common.

Management includes elucidating the underlying cause and symptoms are treated by the insertion of a stent under radiological control in the compressed vena cava. Anticoagulation is also required to prevent clot formation in the stent. The expandable stent usually relieves symptoms within 24 hours. Radiotherapy can also relieve symptoms. The underlying cause should be treated. In this case the lung tumour is inoperable and the prognosis is poor.

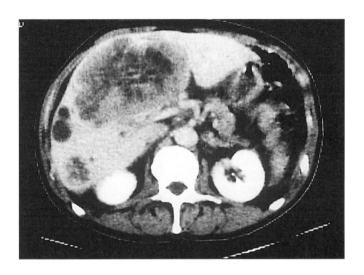

Questions

This 68-year-old man presented with a history of rectal bleeding and weight loss. His investigations included blood tests and a barium enema. As a result of the abnormal liver function tests he had CT of the abdomen and pelvis.

a. What does the CT scan show?
b. What is the underlying diagnosis?
c. What is the management?

Answers

a. The CT showed that the man had extensive liver metastases seen as low attenuation areas.

b. Colonic cancer.

c. The management in this case is mainly palliative as this patient has extensive liver metastases. This may include laser therapy to prevent rectal bleeding and a bypass operation (e.g. colostomy) to prevent intestinal obstruction.

Discussion

In this case the metastases are too extensive for resection. In some cases of liver metastases from a colonic primary a cure can still be obtained by resection of a segment or segments of the liver. This requires a solitary or small number of metastases in such a position that they can be resected, leaving the rest of the liver in situ. If such surgery is being considered it is very important to accurately demonstrate the number of metastases present and their relationship to the segmental anatomy of the liver. CT or MRI are used in such cases with contrast enhancement.

The CT scan was to stage the tumour both locally and to exclude liver metastases, especially in view of the abnormal liver function tests. If this question alone was all that one wanted to know then ultrasound might have been sufficient.

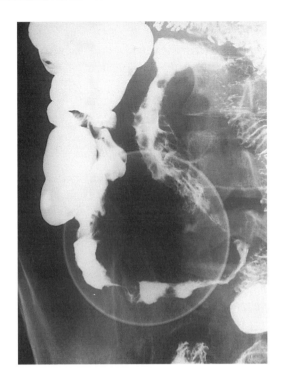

Questions

This 25-year-old Caucasian smoker presented with a history of right iliac fossa pain and weight loss. A mass was palpable in the right iliac fossa. Blood tests revealed anaemia and elevated serum C-reactive protein.

a. What examination is this?
b. What does it show?
c. What is the diagnosis?

Answers

a. The film shows the terminal ileum and caecum from a barium small bowel study (follow through).

b. The distal ileum is markedly distorted, oedematous and ulcerated.

c. In a Caucasian the diagnosis is that of Crohn's disease (in Asians TB should be considered).

Discussion

Crohn's disease is commoner in Caucasians than in Afro-Caribbean people and is much more common in smokers (while ulcerative colitis is mainly a disease of non-smokers).

The ileocaecal region is the most common site affected, followed by the colon and ileum. The patient usually presents with intermittent abdominal pain, diarrhoea and abdominal distension. There may be anaemia, weight loss due to malabsorption and the passage of blood PR. Mouth ulceration and perianal fistulae and sepsis are quite common (20% of cases). There may be uveitis, arthritis and skin rashes (erythema nodosum and pyoderma gangrenosum). Renal stones are more common (10% of cases). Histologically Crohn's disease is a granulomatous inflammatory disorder of the intestine but any part of the gastrointestinal tract can be involved. Classically short lengths of the intestine are involved ('skip lesions'). Management includes:

- Stopping smoking (reduces the risk of recurrence)
- Dietary therapy
- Corticosteroids (short term)
- Surgery
- 5-aminosalicylates (maintenance therapy, but less effective in Crohn's disease than in ulcerative colitis)
- Azathioprine or methotrexate (not long term)
- Metronidazole (not long term).

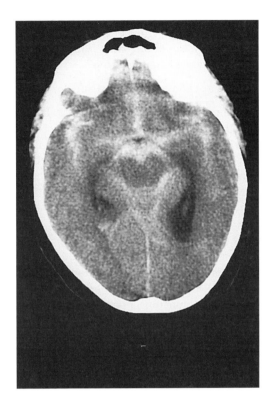

Questions

This 32-year-old woman was admitted as an emergency with a history of sudden onset of severe headache. There was no past history of note and she was usually in good health.

a. What abnormality is shown on this slice on the CT brain scan?
b. What is the diagnosis?
c. List two other symptoms she may have.

Answers

a. The normal black CSF seen in the basal cisterns and sylvian fissures is replaced by white, representing fresh blood.

b. The appearance is that of a subarachnoid haemorrhage.

c. Photophobia, vomiting, neck stiffness, diplopia (if associated with a cranial nerve palsy, a third cranial nerve palsy can be caused by a posterior communicating artery aneurysm or a sixth cranial nerve palsy may be due to raised intracranial pressure), hemiplegia due to cerebral infarction which can be associated with a subarachnoid haemorrhage, due to vasospasm.

Discussion

The berry aneurysm which is usually responsible is rarely seen on a CT scan. It is better demonstrated by carotid arteriography or magnetic resonance angiography (MRA), although the latter will miss small aneurysms. The aneurysms occur at branching points of the intracranial arteries. The commonest sites are the anterior communicating artery, the posterior communicating artery and the middle cerebral artery. Other causes include arteriovenous malformations and trauma. A subarachnoid haemorrhage carries with it a substantial morbidity and mortality. The mortality is from the haemorrhage and associated cerebral infarction. Cerebral ischaemia in infarction can be limited by the drug nimodipine which should be prescribed in all cases. The patient should initially receive supportive therapy with intravenous fluids, oxygen and analgesia. All cases of subarachnoid haemorrhage should be discussed early with a neurosurgeon as early surgical intervention may be necessary to prevent further bleeding. The risks of surgery in some cases may outweigh the benefits.

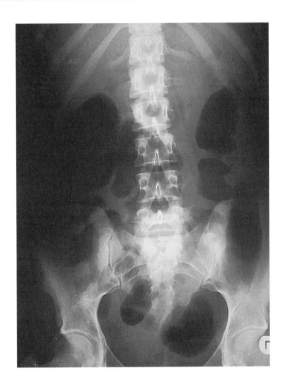

Questions

This 30-year-old woman presented with abdominal pain and bloody diarrhoea with generalized malaise and weight loss. Her mother suffered from similar problems but also had chronic arthritis and a skin rash.

a. What does this plain abdominal film show?
b. What is the most likely diagnosis?
c. What type of arthritis does her mother have?
d. What is the HLA association?

Answers

a. The mucosal pattern of the entire large bowel is abnormal. The appearance of 'thumbprinting' of its wall indicates oedema. The patient therefore has a pancolitis.

b. Ulcerative colitis is the most likely diagnosis.

c. Psoriatic arthritis.

d. HLA B27.

Discussion

The most likely diagnosis is ulcerative colitis as the whole colon is involved whereas in Crohn's disease 'skip' lesions are more common. In a severe attack there may be evidence of toxic megacolon on the plain abdominal film where there is marked dilatation of the large bowel and this may perforate which is associated with a high mortality. There is a higher incidence of inflammatory bowel disease in patients with seronegative arthropathies (e.g. psoriasis, Reiter's disease, ankylosing spondylitis, Behçet's syndrome). These seronegative spondarthritides, as they are known, are associated with HLA B27 and Behçet's syndrome is also associated with HLA B5.

Ulcerative colitis may present in the same clinical manner as Crohn's disease but histologically there are no granulomas. There is chronic inflammatory cell infiltration of the lamina propria and reduction of goblet cells. The large intestine is involved in a continuous manner, usually beginning in the rectum, and the entire colon may be involved. Pseudopolyps are common. There is an increased incidence of colonic carcinoma in these patients (after about 10 years of the disease). Non-colonic complications include:

- **Skin rashes**. Erythema nodosum, pyoderma gangrenosum, leg ulcers (2% of cases)
- **Arthropathy**. This involves the large joints, sacroileitis and ankylosing spondylitis (15% of cases)
- **Liver disease**. Chronic active hepatitis, fatty infiltration, ascending cholangitis. Cirrhosis and cholangiocarcinoma
- **Eyes**. Iritis, episcleritis (5% of cases)
- **Deep vein thrombosis**
- **Secondary amyloidosis**.

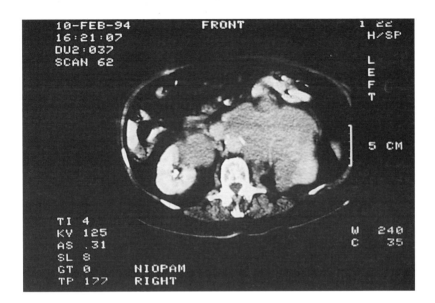

```
10-FEB-94          FRONT                    1 ⊏⊏
16:21:07                                    H⁄SP
DU2:037                                     L
SCAN 62                                     E
                                            F
                                            T

                                            5 CM

TI 4
KV 125
AS .31
SL 8                                        W    240
GT 0      NIOPAM                            C     35
TP 177    RIGHT
```

Questions

This 70-year-old man presented with weight loss and night sweats.

a. What does this enhanced contrast CT of the abdomen show?
b. What is the likely diagnosis?

Answers

a. There is a lobulated soft tissue mass extending from the para-aortic area towards both kidneys. This is extensive lymphadenopathy

b. The most likely diagnosis in a man of this age with these symptoms is non-Hodgkin's lymphoma. Hodgkin's lymphoma is a possibility but usually this presents in younger (30–40 years) men. Other possibilities would include lymphadenopathy due to spread from other primary tumours (e.g. kidney) and also infection (e.g. tuberculosis) should be excluded but these differential diagnoses are less likely. The pattern here is strongly in favour of lymphoma.

Discussion

It is essential to obtain tissue for a histological diagnosis. This can be done by guided biopsy under CT scan control. The patient may have more accessible lymph nodes (e.g. supraclavicular) for biopsy. Other investigations required include chest X-ray, full blood count, electrolytes, liver function tests, bone marrow examination.

The clinical staging of lymphoma depends upon which lymph node areas are involved and also the presence of symptoms known as B symptoms, i.e. weight loss, fever. The absence of symptoms is known as class A. The regional lymphadenopathy classification is as follows:

I   A single lymph node region (usually one side of the neck)
II   Two regions involved on the same side of the diaphragm
III Lymph node regions involved above and below the diaphragm but limited to lymph nodes or spleen involvement (liver involvement excluded)
IV   Widespread involvement including bone marrow, liver and other tissues (e.g. lung, skin).

The case described is at least IB.

CT of the chest, abdomen and pelvis is used in initial staging and in the follow-up after chemotherapy. In NHL involvement of different nodal groups may involve non-contiguous areas, while Hodgkin's disease is contiguous in its pattern of involvement.

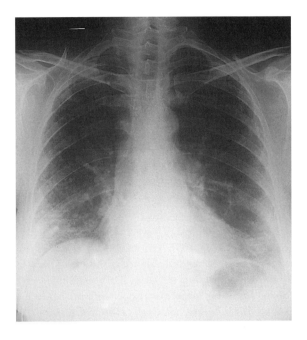

Questions

This 60-year-old woman presented with a history of progressively worsening shortness of breath and non-productive cough.

a. What abnormality does the chest radiograph show?
b. What is the most likely diagnosis?
c. List two clinical signs which may be present.
d. What will her lung function tests show?

Answers

a. There is reticular (linear) shadowing at both lung bases. This represents fibrosis.

b. The most likely cause is cryptogenic fibrosing alveolitis (CFA).

c. Finger clubbing, late fine inspiratory crackles on auscultation of the chest, central cyanosis, dyspnoea, poor chest expansion.

d. Her lung function tests will show a restrictive defect with an FEV1/FVC%>70%. The transfer factor is reduced.

Discussion

The combination of the clinical picture and the radiological appearance, especially on high resolution CT scan of the lungs makes the diagnosis. Lung biopsy is now rarely needed. The distribution of the fibrosis makes cryptogenic fibrosing alveolitis the most likely diagnosis but this appearance is seen in fibrosing alveolitis associated with other causes which must be excluded. These are collagen vascular diseases (e.g. scleroderma, rheumatoid arthritis), asbestosis (usually pleural plaques and thickening are evident on the film), drugs (amiodarone, nitrofurantoin, busulphan). The reticular shadowing can progress to honeycombing and spread throughout the lungs. There can be associated volume loss but often there is compensatory development of upper lobe emphysema which maintains the lung volume.

CT can not only make the diagnosis but can also help to show the relative amounts of established fibrosis and active inflammation. In the early inflammatory phase, treatment with corticosteroids and cyclophosphamide can result in improvement. When the pattern is predominantly one of fibrosis, however, this has no effect. The prognosis of CFA is poor with only a 50% 5 year survival rate. There is also an increased risk of lung carcinoma.

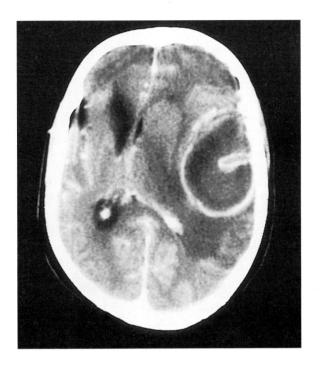

Questions

This 39-year-old had recently complained of headaches but is now confused and drowsy. There is right-sided weakness on examination and he has papilloedema.

a. What abnormality does this enhanced CT of the brain show?
b. Give a differential diagnosis.
c. What is the most likely diagnosis?

Answers

a. A cystic mass in the left parietal lobe.

b. Abscess or glioma.

c. Cerebral abscess.

Discussion

There is a ring enhancing mass in the left parietal lobe with surrounding oedema. This is producing compression of the ipsilateral lateral ventricle. Such a lesion could represent a cerebral abscess, a glioma or possibly a metastasis. The thin smooth wall is more in favour of an abscess (as was indeed the case). In the early stages only cerebritis is seen. This appears as oedema and some contrast enhancement may be seen. After about 10 days capsule formation is present. A brain abscess may arise from infection in adjacent structures (especially the middle ear or frontal sinuses), via haematogenous spread (in patients with cyanotic congenital heart disease, lung abscess or bronchiectasis, though the latter is less common now) and sometimes following penetrating injury or surgery. The CT brain scan will also show any opacification of the sinuses, middle ear or mastoids. A chest radiograph should reveal any pulmonary source of infection or cardiac disease. However, the clinical examination would be expected to reveal middle ear infection or cardiorespiratory disease.

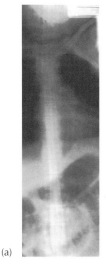

(a)

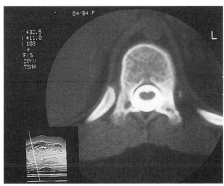

(b)

Questions

This child presents with leg weakness and enuresis.

a. What examinations are shown in Figures a and b?
b. What do they show?
c. What investigation has largely replaced these in such cases?

Answers

a. A myelogram and CT myelogram.

b. Diastematomyelia.

c. MRI.

Discussion

Figure a is a film from a myelogram. A water-soluble contrast medium has been injected into the thecal sac and is outlining the spinal cord. Figure b is an axial CT slice of the spine obtained while the myelographic contrast is present. The contrast is seen as white. Both these investigations have now largely been replaced by MRI except where this cannot be performed because of severe claustrophobia or contraindications such as the presence of berry aneurysm clips, a cardiac pacemaker, some types of cardiac valve replacement, cochlear implants, intraocular metallic foreign bodies, etc. In Figure a contrast is seen in a vertically running cleft in the cord. The CT myelogram (Fig. b) shows the cord starting to divide into two. This condition is diastematomyelia. It is often associated with other types of spinal dysraphism such as cord tethering, myelomeningocele and lipomyelomeningocele. There are two types of diastematomyelia: one where the cords lie in the same thecal sac and another where the thecal sac is divided into two by a vertically running septum of bone, cartilage or fibrous tissue. Imaging can show the extent of the diastem and, more importantly, whether the cord reunites at its lower end.

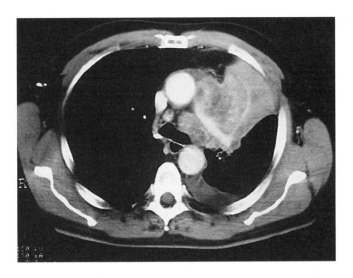

Questions

This CT scan of the chest was performed on a 67-year-old man.

a. What does it show?
b. What is the diagnosis?
c. What question is CT asked to answer in this condition?

Answers

a. A left hilar mass.

b. Lung cancer.

c. Confirm the presence of a mass seen on the chest radiograph and stage the tumour.

Discussion

There is a mass surrounding the left pulmonary artery which is narrowed as a result. The mass shows irregular enhancement with the intravenous contrast medium. In addition the left upper lobe shows consolidation and some collapse. A pleural effusion is also seen. The diagnosis is that of primary lung carcinoma. In such cases CT is useful to confirm the presence of a mass and to stage the carcinoma. One needs to assess the site and size of the primary tumour and any chest wall or mediastinal structure invasion. Also any lymph node enlargement or metastases should be commented upon. Hence the scan covers the chest and liver. Lymph node involvement is difficult as nodes are assessed purely on size criteria. A short axis diameter of over 1 cm is considered abnormal but not all involved nodes are enlarged and some enlarged nodes are just reactive in nature rather than involved with tumour. The larger the node the more likely it is to be malignant. The CT stage of the tumour is then given using the TNM classification. This information is then taken along with the clinical and bronchoscopic data when assessing whether the tumour is operable for cure. Some have cast doubt on the value of CT staging because of the problem with judging lymphadenopathy. None the less, it is still widely performed. Before operability is decided the patient may also need a CT scan of his head and an isotope bone scan to exclude metastases. This practice is not universal, however, and the pick up rate of unsuspected lesions is low.

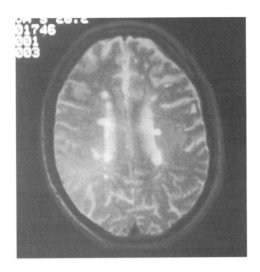

Questions

This is a T2-weighted axial slice from an MRI scan of the brain of a 30-year-old woman.

a. What abnormality is shown?
b. What is the most likely diagnosis?
c. What other conditions could cause this appearance?

Answers

a. Multiple areas of high signal (white density) lesions in the white matter.

b. Multiple sclerosis (MS).

c. Infarcts; usually due to vasculitic conditions such as systemic lupus erythematosus (SLE) in this age group.

Discussion

Multiple small areas of high signal (appearing white) are seen in the white matter, especially around the lateral ventricles. In a patient of this age with an appropriate history the most likely diagnosis is multiple sclerosis. MRI is the imaging modality of choice in MS and can show plaques in the brain and spinal cord. Small infarcts can also cause similar areas of high signal on T2-weighted scans. Usually this is seen in an older age group of patients, except if there is a cause of vasculitis such as SLE. MS plaques often have their long axis at right angles to the lateral ventricles which can help in differentiation. The clinical presentation is also important, as are the demonstration of delayed visually evoked responses and oligoclonal bands of IgG in the cerebrospinal fluid (CSF). MS is a disease of unknown aetiology that causes plaques of demyelination throughout the central nervous system. There is an association with HLA B7 and HLA DRW2. It may present with retrobulbar neuritis, sensory or motor disturbances depending on plaque location. The commonest presentation is with upper motor neurone deficit, (hemiparesis, monoparesis or paraparesis). There may be sensory deficit with paraesthesiae and/or loss of position sense. Cerebellar signs are common, (nystagmus, dysarthria, intention tremor, past pointing, dysdiadochokinesia, pendular reflexes). Diplopia due to internuclear paralysis and ataxic nystagmus (nystagmus more pronounced in the abducting eye) are common. Other clinical features include: vertigo, vomiting, disturbed micturition, mood changes (depressions, euphoria, dementia). Symptoms are often made worse by exertion and heat. Hence the patient may be able to get into a hot bath but be unable to get out (Utoff's sign). The course may vary from complete recovery from the first episode to one of relentless deterioration. Approximately 80% have a relapsing/remitting illness that often then becomes progressive. Poor prognostic features include: motor or cerebellar lesions, onset in 20s, or recurrence within 6 months of presentation; males have a poorer outcome than females. Treatment of patients with relapsing disease with interferon-β-1A has been shown to reduce exacerbation rate and may slow the progression of disability.

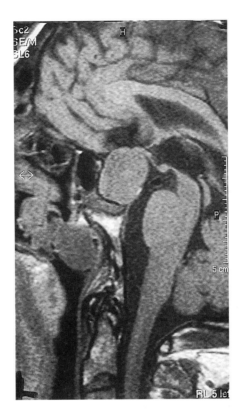

Questions

This 30-year-old woman complains of galactorrhoea.

a. What is this examination?
b. What does it show?
c. What occular abnormality may be detectable on examining the patient?

Answers

a. MRI scan of the pituitary (sagittal midline slice).

b. A pituitary adenoma.

c. A visual field defect: bitemporal hemianopia.

Discussion

This is an image from an MRI scan of the pituitary. It is a sagittal midline slice with T1 weighting. The main abnormality demonstrated is a macroadenoma of the pituitary which extends superiorly out of the pituitary fossa. Such a pituitary tumour could compress the optic chiasm, leading to bitemporal hemianopia. The optic chiasm is easier to assess on coronal images, which would also be performed. MRI is the imaging modality of choice for suspected pituitary tumours. T1-weighted images are best and in most cases gadolinium enhancement adds little to the information obtained from unenhanced images. In many cases no adenoma can be resolved even when hormone levels are raised. This patient has a prolactinoma. These tumours cause galactorrhoea and infertility in the female and glactorrhoea and impotence in the male. Hyperprolactinaemia can also be caused by drugs (e.g. oestrogens, domperidone, tranquillizers). Treatment can be surgical but usually bromocriptine (a dopamine agonist) is prescribed first.

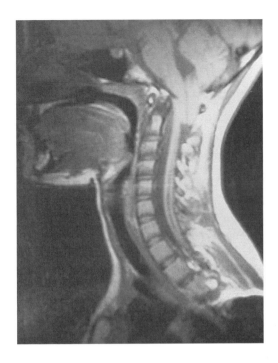

Questions

This is the image of a 30-year-old patient with loss of pain and temperature sensation in the upper limbs and weakness and muscle wasting in the hands.

a. Give two abnormalities seen.
b. What type of scan is this?

Answers

a. ● *Arnold–Chiari malformation
   ● A syrinx in the cervical spinal cord.

b. A sagittal mid-line slice from a T1-weighted MRI scan.

Discussion

There is herniation of the cerebellar tonsils through the foramen magnum and the syrinx is shown as low attenuation within the spinal cord. This is a Chiari type I malformation, the mildest of the four types originally described by Chiari. There is usually no hydrocephalus in this form. The Chiari II malformation is more complex with most patients presenting in the neonatal period. It is very common in patients with myelomeningocele and encephalocele and is often associated with spina bifida. There is hydrocephalus and early shunting of this is important. Medullary compression is another feature and can be life threatening. Syringomyelia is the commonest cause of neuropathic joints in the upper limbs. It affects the spinothalamic tracts (pain and temperature sensation) which cross centrally in the spinal cord, rather than the posterior columns (touch and proprioception) which remain ipsilateral at this level (crossing at a higher level in the medulla). It also causes muscle wasting and weakness of the upper limbs, especially the hands. Symptoms may start unilaterally. As well as idiopathic cases and those associated with a Chiari malformation, a syrinx can be secondary to trauma or a spinal cord tumour.

---

*J. Arnold (1835–1915), German pathologist. H. Chiari (1851–1916), Austrian pathologist.

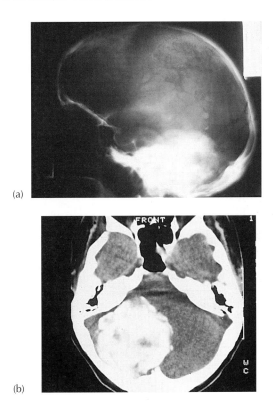

(a)

(b)

Questions

This 65-year-old lady complained of some loss of balance. She was mildly ataxic with a broad-based gait and other cerebellar signs detectable on examination.

a. What abnormality is shown on this lateral skull radiograph?
b. What is the most likely cause for this?
c. What further investigation is shown?

Answers

a. A sclerotic area in the posterior cranial fossa.

b. Meningioma.

c. CT of the brain.

Discussion

The large area of sclerosis in the posterior fossa represents calcification and it is most likely to be a meningioma. They often calcify and can also produce a sclerotic reaction in overlying bone. A meningioma is a benign tumour (though malignant change can occur). The next examination in this case would be either CT or MRI. The latter would just show a single void due to the marked calcification. The CT examination can be seen. Depending on their size, location and the clinical picture, treatment of a meningioma can be with surgery, radiotherapy or just adopting a follow-up programme with no treatment. In this case the tumour is large and is compressing the cerebellum, brain stem and fourth ventricle so surgical treatment is required.

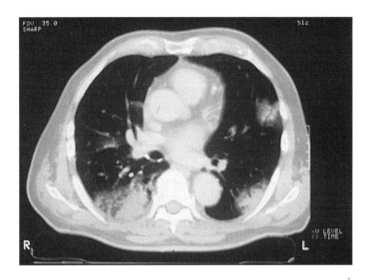

Questions

This is a slice from a CT scan of the chest performed on a 65-year-old patient with a history of weight loss and a cough productive of frothy white sputum.

a. What abnormality is shown?
b. Give three possible causes for this appearance.
c. Which is the most likely in this case?

Answers

a. Peripheral areas of consolidation with air bronchograms.

b. ● Pneumonia (infective, usually bacterial)
   ● Eosinophilic pneumonia
   ● Alveolar cell carcinoma
   ● Sarcoidosis.

c. Alveolar cell carcinoma.

Discussion

Consolidation can be just due to simple infection, or where there are several peripheral areas eosinophilic pneumonia should be considered. In this condition the consolidation is typically flitting in nature with new areas developing as others resolve. Pseudoalveolar sarcoid can also be a cause of such areas of consolidation. Alveolar cell carcinoma is one of the histological types of lung cancer. Others are: squamous cell carcinoma (40%), small cell carcinoma (25%), large cell carcinoma (20%); the remainder are adenocarinomas (15%) and alveolar cell carcinomas are rarer. An alveolar cell carcinoma can appear as a lung mass or as one or more areas of consolidation. A whole lobe may be infiltrated with tumour or, like transitional cell carcinoma of the urothelium, there may be multiple primaries. It is a variant of adenocarcinoma.

Clinically there will be reduced expansion bilaterally with reduced air entry and areas of bronchial breathing. There will be dullness to percussion. Typical symptoms of consolidation are: dyspnoea, cough, haemoptysis and pleurisy. It is important that infection (particularly atypical) is excluded by sputum and blood culture and plasma serology. Bronchoscopy and biopsy as well as sputum cytology should confirm the diagnosis histologically.

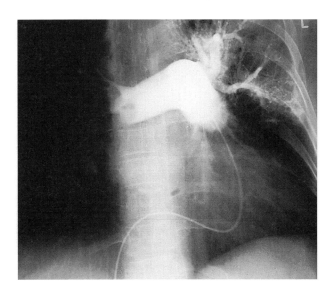

Questions

This 46-year-old patient presented with sudden onset of bilateral pleuritic chest pain, and shortness of breath.

a. What examination is this?
b. What abnormalities are seen?
c. What is the diagnosis?
d. What other symptoms may she have (list two)?

Answers

a. A pulmonary arteriogram.

b. Absent perfusion to the left lower lobe and the whole right lung with filling defects within the vessels.

c. Pulmonary thromboembolism.

d. Haemoptysis, palpitations, dizziness, syncope (the last two are due to decreased cardiac output and reduced cerebral perfusion).

Discussion

Pulmonary embolism (PE) is usually secondary to thrombus in the deep veins of the lower limbs or pelvis. Initial investigation of a suspected PE is with a chest radiograph and radioisotope ventilation perfusion lung scan. This is reported as being normal, or showing low, intermediate/indeterminate or high probability of pulmonary embolism. The intermediate/ indeterminate probability classification is particularly common in patients with chronic obstructive pulmonary disease. The radiological and clinical probabilities are both taken into account in making a diagnosis. Where one is left unsure, further investigation can be with spiral CT or conventional pulmonary arteriography or with venography or Doppler ultrasound of the leg veins to give corroborative evidence. Treatment is with anticoagulation, initially with heparin (low molecular weight heparin is now used) and then warfarin for 6 months. In this case, however, the embolism is so extensive that thrombolysis or embolectomy may be required. That was the reason for the arteriogram in this case. Usually such large emboli result in collapse and sudden death. The mortality is high (about 30%) even with treatment.

Predisposing factors for deep vein thrombosis and subsequent pulmonary emboli include:

- Underlying carcinoma
- Prolonged immobility (e.g. following stroke, myocardial infarction etc.)
- Postoperative (especially after pelvic surgery) (classically occurs at 10th postoperative day)
- Oral contraceptive pill/pregancy
- Hyperviscosity syndromes (e.g. polycythaemia rubra vera, Waldenström's macroglobulinaemia).

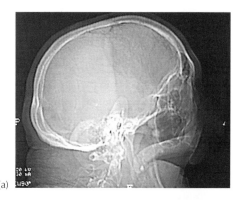

(a)

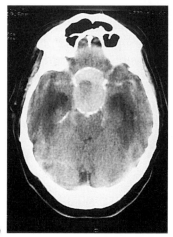

(b)

Questions

This 60-year-old woman presented with headaches.

a. What abnormality is shown on the lateral skull radiograph (Fig. a)?
b. Give two abnormalities seen on the contrast enhanced CT scan (Fig. b).
c. What is the diagnosis?
d. What complication has developed?

Answers

a. Enlargement of the pituitary fossa.

b. • An enhancing mass in the region of the pituitary fossa
   • Dilatation of the temporal horns of the lateral ventricle.

c. A pituitary tumour (adenoma).

d. Hydrocephalus.

Discussion

Most pituitary tumours are too small to resolve on imaging, even on MRI which is now the investigation of choice. A large tumour, however, will enlarge the pituitary fossa with erosion of its floor and the posterior clinoid processes. Extension superiorly out of the fossa can result in the adenoma pressing on the optic chiasm which lies directly above the pituitary fossa. This will result in bitemporal hemianopia as the nerves responsible for the temporal parts of the visual fields cross at this point. Further enlargement, as here, compresses the third ventricle causing hydrocephalus of the lateral ventricles. Pituitary tumours can be non-functioning or secrete hormones, especially prolactin or growth hormone (the latter causing acromegaly in adults). Therefore their hormonal effects may be due to over or under production of the various pituitary hormones. This large tumour will need to be removed surgically as it is causing pressure effects. Preoperatively the patient's pituitary function should be checked and corrected appropriately.

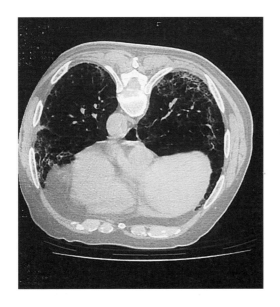

Questions

This 50-year-old lady is known to have rheumatoid arthritis. She complains of worsening shortness of breath.

a. What examination is this?
b. What does it show?
c. What is the diagnosis?
d. What will her pulmonary function tests show?

Answers

a. High resolution CT of the lungs.

b. Posterior basal pulmonary fibrosis.

c. Fibrosing alveolitis.

d. A restrictive defect and reduced transfer factor.

Discussion

Fibrosing alveolitis is a well recognized association with collagen vascular diseases such as rheumatoid arthritis. It is particularly common in systemic sclerosis. Similar pulmonary changes are seen in cryptogenic fibrosing alveolitis, asbestosis and as a complication of some drugs (e.g. nitrofurantoin, amiodarone, penicillamine and various cytotoxic drugs such as busulphan, bleomycin, vincristine and methotrexate). The disease starts at the posterior lung bases and early changes can be confused with a gravity dependent artefact often seen at this site on high resolution CT. The distinction can be made as in this case by turning the patient prone. The artefact will move but genuine pathology remains unchanged. The prognosis is poor, especially in cryptogenic fibrosing alveolitis which has a 50% 5 year survival rate. Its cause is unknown but smoking seems to be important in triggering the disease. The early inflammatory phase of the disease can be seen on CT as ground-glass shadowing. At this stage treatment with steroids and cyclophosphamide results in some improvement. However, once the picture is one of predominant fibrosis (as in this case) treatment is often less successful.

Clinically the most distressing symptom is breathlessness. The patient has a dry cough and wheeze is uncommon. Signs include: finger clubbing, cyanosis, reduced chest expansion and basal fine, late inspiratory crackles. There may be signs of consolidation (bronchial breathing, dullness to percussion). The mainstay of treatment is with steroids, home oxygen and antibiotics for intercurrent infections. The course of the condition is progressive and the patient ultimately develops respiratory failure.

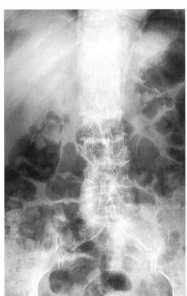

(a)

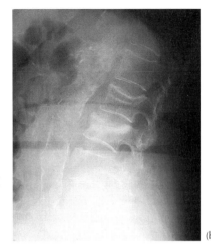

(b)

Questions

This 75-year-old woman complains of back pain which came on suddenly a few weeks before these films were taken.

a. What abnormality is seen on the radiographs of her lumbar spine?
b. What is the likely underlying cause?
c. What two other causes would you consider?

Answers

a. Compression fractures of the vertebral bodies of L2 and L3.

b. Osteoporosis.

c. ● Myeloma
   ● Metastases.

Discussion

Osteoporotic vertebral collapse is common in post-menopausal women, in the elderly in general, and in patients on corticosteroids. Such fractures can occur even in the absence of trauma. These groups of patients are also prone to other fractures elsewhere, most notably a *Colles' fracture and fracture of the femoral neck. The latter is a major cause of morbidity and mortality in the elderly. Plain films show generalized osteopenia although it is not possible to specifically diagnose osteoporosis from a radiograph. The fact that the pedicles of the vertebrae are still intact is a little against the presence of metastases but this does not exclude myeloma which can produce generalized osteopenia as well as more focal lytic lesions. Even MRI cannot fully distinguish osteoporotic collapse from underlying malignancy, though it does have a higher specificity than plain films. In this case there is some sign of healing as evidenced by the sclerosis. Development of osteoporosis in post-menopausal women is delayed by a large mineralized bone mass in earlier life, helped by a high intake of dairy products, for example, and by exercise. Hormone replacement therapy also delays bone loss. Treatment of osteoporosis can be with calcium supplements and biphosphonates.

---

*A. Colles (1773–1843), Irish surgeon.

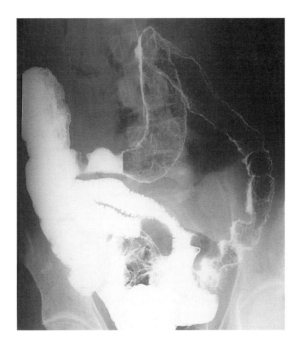

Questions

This 35-year-old man presented with diarrhoea and rectal bleeding. He also complained of blurred vision.

a. What does this barium enema show?
b. What is the diagnosis?
c. What skin lesion may he have?
d. What is the likely cause of his blurred vision?

Answers

a. The large bowel is markedly abnormal with mucosal ulceration present.

b. Ulcerative colitis.

c. Erythema nodosum, pyoderma gangrenosum. Psoriasis is more common.

d. Uveitis or iritis.

Discussion

Although ulcerative colitis (UC) and Crohn's disease are both classed as inflammatory bowel diseases, they manifest themselves very differently. Ulcerative colitis only involves the large bowel while Crohn's disease can affect anywhere from the mouth to the anus. UC is seen to involve the rectum and extend proximally in continuity, while Crohn's often spares the rectum and is characterized by skip lesions. UC is a disease that causes ulceration of the mucosa/submucosa but Crohn's disease produces transmural inflammation, hence fistulae are not a feature of UC. UC does have a range of complications outside the bowel such as arthritis, uveitis, episcleritis, sclerosing cholangitis and cholangiocarcinoma. Most, though not of course all, of these regress after colectomy which also cures the ulcerative colitis. Crohn's, however, cannot be cured by surgery. The features in this case that indicate the diagnosis of UC rather than Crohn's disease are the rectal bleeding (common in UC but unusual in Crohn's disease), continuous involvement from the rectum proximally, sparing of the terminal ileum, and superficial ulceration. In an acute attack of UC it is important to be alert for the development of toxic colitis that can progress to megacolon and perforation. This, and massive haemorrhage, are indications for emergency surgery. The mortality is high (up to 50%) in these cases. Surgery is also used more electively in some cases of UC where medical control with 5-aminosalicylates and corticosteroids has failed, or where malignancy has developed (the incidence of large bowel carcinoma starts to rise after 8–10 years of the disease). Malignancy is more a problem with UC than with Crohn's disease. In UC a stricture should be considered as likely to be malignant, while in Crohn's disease benign strictures are a typical feature.

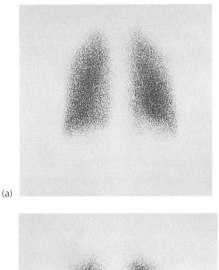

(a)

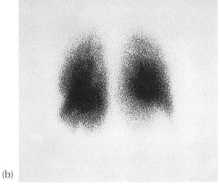

(b)

Questions

This 32-year-old woman presented with a sudden onset of breathlessness and pleuritic chest pain.

a. What are these investigations?
b. What abnormality is demonstrated?
c. What is the diagnosis?

Answers

a. Ventilation (a) and perfusion (b) isotope lungs scans.

b. Multiple perfusion defects with a normal ventilation scan.

c. Pulmonary emboli.

Discussion

Pulmonary embolism (PE) is usually secondary to thrombus in the deep veins of the lower limbs or pelvis. The first line investigation is a radio-isotope ventilation perfusion lung scan. A typical case of pulmonary embolism will show multiple segmental perfusion defects with a normal ventilation scan. The result is by no means always a clear yes or no, however. The scan is reported along with a chest radiograph and is assigned to one of the following classifications: normal, low probability, intermediate/indeterminate probability, or high probability. The degree of clinical suspicion is also taken into account. Where both the lung scan and clinical suspicion give a high probability of PE then the patient is anticoagulated with low dose heparin and warfarin, and where both suggest a low probability another diagnosis must be considered. However, this still leaves a significant number of patients where there is uncertainty. This is especially a problem in patients with chronic obstructive pulmonary disease where the lung scan will be classed as indeterminate probability. In these cases one needs to resort to further imaging. The choices are pulmonary arteriography, a spiral CT pulmonary arteriogram, or the imaging of leg veins with colour flow Doppler ultrasound or venography to look for a deep venous thrombosis (DVT). Indeed, in patients with chronic obstructive pulmonary disease, it is probably best to proceed directly to a spiral CT pulmonary angiogram as the radioisotope lung scan will give an indeterminate result anyway. Spiral CT has the advantage over conventional pulmonary arteriography in that it is non-invasive (the latter requires introducing a catheter into the pulmonary arteries via the femoral vein and the right side of the heart). The spiral CT angiogram is as accurate as conventional pulmonary angiography down to the segmental level and only misses the 6% of cases of pulmonary embolism which are purely subsegmental in distribution.

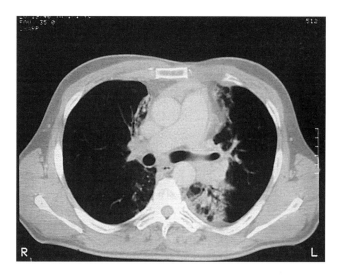

Questions

This 65-year-old man is complaining of increasing shortness of breath. He has previously received treatment for adenocarcinoma.

a. What abnormality is seen on this CT scan of the chest?
b. What is the diagnosis?

Answers

a. Fibrosis and consolidation in the medial aspects of both lungs.

b. Radiation pneumonitis/fibrosis. He has had mediastinal radiotherapy.

Discussion

Damage to normal tissues in the radiotherapy field is an obvious complication of such treatment. In the lung this can result in pneumonitis and the development of fibrosis. It is pneumonitis which produces the most symptoms and this occurs 1–6 months after radiotherapy. There is associated arteritis. Changes progress to fibrosis and the patient can also develop progressive sclerosis of the pulmonary vessels which can result in lung damage more peripherally, outside the radiation field. There can also be damage to the bronchi which may lead to bronchiectasis. In this case the areas of abnormality in both lungs have a straight lateral margin corresponding to the edge of the radiation field. This demarcation does not correspond to any normal lung anatomy and is diagnostic of radiotherapy induced damage. Radiation may also cause pleural or pericardial effusions, cardiac muscle or coronary artery damage, damage to the oesophagus resulting in dysmotility, strictures or fistulae, and bone damage leading to necrosis. Bone necrosis produces mixed changes with some increased lucency and some sclerosis and non-healing fractures may also occur on occasions.

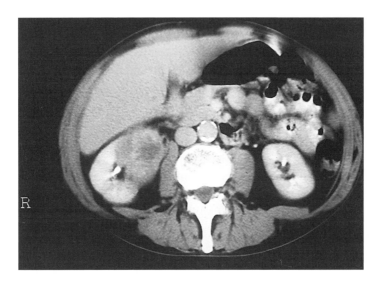

Questions

This 48-year-old man presented with haematuria. Blood tests revealed polycythaemia.

a. What abnormality is seen on this CT scan?
b. What is the diagnosis?
c. What is the reason for his polycythaemia?

Answers

a. A mass in the right kidney.

b. Renal cell carcinoma.

c. Excess erythropoietin secretion by the tumour.

Discussion

Haematuria is a common problem and can be due to a range of different conditions such as renal cell or transitional cell carcinoma, benign or malignant prostatic disease, infection, calculi, etc. Tests would include a full blood count and urea and electrolyte levels, urine cytology and possibly cystoscopy. Radiological investigation can start with either ultrasound or an intravenous urogram (IVU). If the first of these is negative one has to proceed to the other. The IVU is superior for renal or bladder calculi and for transitional cell carcinoma of the urothelium. Ultrasound shows renal cell carcinoma or prostatic enlargement better. If a renal cell carcinoma is discovered then it is staged using CT. This is to show any invasion outside the kidney into the adjacent fat, para-aortic lymphadenopathy, tumour thrombus in the renal vein or inferior vena cava, or the presence of metastases (particularly in the liver or lungs). If practicable, treatment is with nephrectomy.

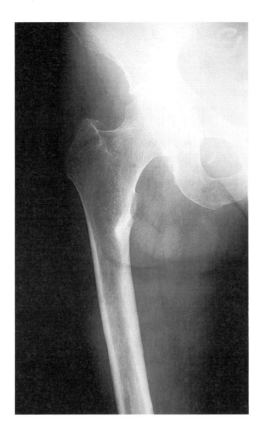

Questions

This 75-year-old woman presented with pain in her right hip. She had difficulty combing her hair.

a. What abnormality is seen on this radiograph of the right hip and upper femur?
b. What name is given to this appearance?
c. What is the diagnosis?
d. What is the reason for her difficulty combing her hair?
e. List two possible biochemical abnormalities.

Answers

a. Below the lesser trochanter on the medial aspect of the upper femoral shaft is a horizontal lucent line with surrounding sclerosis.

b. This is a Looser's zone or Milkman fracture.

c. Osteomalacia.

d. Proximal myopathy. Patients also find it difficult to stand up from sitting and have difficulty going upstairs.

e. Hypocalcaemia, hypophosphataemia, raised alkaline phosphatase.

Discussion

Osteomalacia ('adult rickets') is due to vitamin D deficiency or a problem in its metabolism. Vitamin D_3 synthesized in the skin or taken in as part of the diet is hydroxylated in the liver with a second hydroxylation step in the kidneys. Osteomalacia may therefore result from a problem with synthesis in the skin (e.g. Asians in northern latitudes), poor diet, conditions that lead to malabsorption, disturbance of liver function by some anticonvulsant drugs (e.g. phenytoin) and renal disease (including renal osteodystrophy). The biochemistry depends on the cause of the osteomalacia and the stage of the disease. Vitamin D deficiency/malabsorption results in a low serum level of calcium and phosphate with low urine calcium and raised alkaline phosphatase levels (due to increased osteoblastic activity). The hypocalcaemia stimulates parathyroid hormone production, correcting the low calcium but increasing the hypophosphataemia. The bone abnormality in osteomalacia is defective mineralization of osteoid. Osteomalacia responds well to treatment with vitamin D. Looser's zones (pseudo fractures) are one of the radiological features of osteomalacia. They are often symmetrical in the femoral necks and other long bones, pubic rami, scapulae and ribs. They can progress to true fractures. Other findings can include osteopenia, intracortical bone reabsorption due to secondary hyperparathyroidism and bone softening leading to bowing, protrusio acetabuli or basilar invagination.

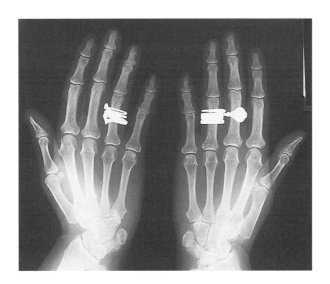

Questions

This 60-year-old woman has difficulty in swallowing and shortness of breath as well as problems with her hands.

a. Give two abnormalities on this radiograph of both hands.
b. What is the diagnosis?

Answers

a. ● Soft tissue loss at the finger tips
   ● Erosion of the tips of the distal phalanges.

b. Systemic sclerosis (scleroderma).

Discussion

Systemic sclerosis is commoner in women than in men. It is part of a range of connective tissue disease. In the hands, in addition to the acro-osteolysis (erosion of the distal phalanges) and soft tissue loss seen here, one can also see soft tissue calcification. The skin is pigmented and tight and vitiligo and telangiectasia may occur. There is often a small oral orifice and a 'beak-shaped' nose. Raynaud's phenomenon is a common presentation. There may be a polyarthropathy similar to rheumatoid arthritis. The effects of systemic sclerosis are more widespread, however, with involvement of the oesophagus, stomach, small bowel and lungs. Pulmonary involvement with a fibrosing alveolitis is common as is aspiration pneumonitis. There is an associated increased incidence of lung cancer. Pulmonary arteritis is also seen in 30% of cases. In the gastro-intestinal tract oesophageal dilatation occurs and also marked gastro-oesophageal reflux. Dilated small bowel with pseudosacculation is also a finding that can be seen on a barium examination. These features are due to loss of smooth muscle in the wall of the oesophagus, stomach and small bowel leading to loss of peristalsis and atonic dilatation. This leads to dysphagia which may also be caused by a peptic oesophageal stricture due to reflux. The small bowel diverticula can lead to bacterial overgrowth and malabsorption. Wide-mouthed diverticula seen on the mesenteric border of the colon on barium enema are typical in systemic sclerosis and contribute to constipation which is common and is also caused by dysmotility. There is cardiac involvement in 50% with myocardial fibrosis, abnormal conduction and cardiomyopathy. Fibrotic pericarditis is also seen, as is renal involvement which leads to hypertension and renal failure. These latter two and/or respiratory failure are the usual terminal events. Treatment is essentially symptomatic. Steroids have no proven value.

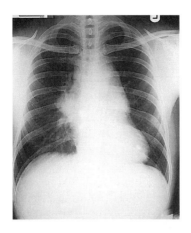

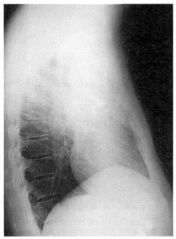

Questions

This 21-year-old man complains of lack of energy and night sweats.

a. What abnormality is seen on the frontal and lateral chest radiographs?
b. What is the cause for this?
c. What is the most likely diagnosis?
d. What may be found on examination?

Answers

a. A lobulated anterior mediastinal mass.

b. Lymphadenopathy.

c. Hodgkin's disease.

d. Anaemia, lymphadenopathy, hepatosplenomegaly.

Discussion

Hodgkin's disease is commoner in men and has two peaks of incidence, one in young adults and a second in the elderly. Its pathological classification is into nodular sclerosing, mixed cellularity, lymphocyte predominant and lymphocyte depleted types. Presentation can be with enlarged nodes (occasionally associated with alcohol-induced pain), fever and night sweats, skin itching, malaise, loss of energy and weight loss. As with other lymphomas it is staged with CT:

- **Stage I**. Only one nodal group involved
- **Stage II**. More than one nodal group involved but limited to one side of the diaphragm
- **Stage III**. Involvement of nodes and/or the spleen on both sides of the diaphragm
- **Stage IV**. Diffuse extra nodal disease.

Unlike non-Hodgkin's lymphoma (NHL), Hodgkin's disease shows contiguous involvement of nodal groups. NHL can involve any nodal groups in no particular pattern. Treatment of Hodgkin's disease is with radiotherapy (stages I or II) or chemotherapy (higher stages). Chemotherapy is based on the original MOPP regime (nitrogen mustard, vincristine, procarbazine, and prednisolone) and its variants (e.g. COPP; cyclophosphamide substituted for nitrogen mustard).

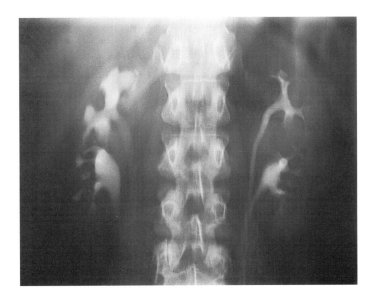

Questions

This 52-year-old woman has had recurrent urinary tract infections.

a. What examination is this?
b. List three abnormalities seen.
c. What is the cause of the abnormalities which are not congenital?

Answers

a. This is a tomogram from an IVU series.

b. ● Bilateral duplex kidneys
   ● Cortical scarring of the right kidney
   ● Calyceal clubbing of the right kidney.

c. The cortical scarring and calyceal clubbing are due to previous pyelonephritis.

Discussion

A duplex system can vary from one where there are two ureters all the way down to the bladder, through ureteric fusion at any point along its length to just a bifid renal pelvis. Often it creates no problems at all and is found incidentally on an IVU done for some other reason. Sometimes, however, it can be associated with obstruction or vesicoureteric reflux. Typically it is the upper moiety that becomes obstructed and the lower one in which reflux occurs. It is the ureter of the upper moiety that has an ectopic insertion. Usually this is just into another part of the bladder, but occasionally it inserts into the urethra below the bladder neck sphincter. In such a situation it is a rare cause of bed wetting in children. Normally the angle of insertion of the ureter into the bladder wall prevents vesicoureteric reflux but when this mechanism does not work children who have urinary infection are at risk of renal damage, the long term sequelae of which are renal scarring and calyceal clubbing as seen here. It is in an attempt to prevent this that children with urinary tract infections are investigated with ultrasound, and, when needed, a micturating cystogram (to show and grade any vesicoureteric reflux), or a radioisotope renogram (to look for renal scarring). Where problems are discovered long term antibiotics are prescribed.

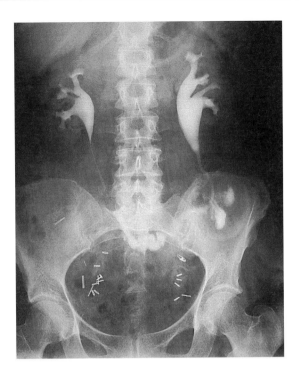

Questions

This IVU was done to investigate haematuria in a 58-year-old woman. No cause was found on the IVU. She had undergone surgery for cancer a year ago.

a. What previous surgery has this patient had?
b. What complications (list two) can occur from such operations?
c. What concern was the IVU to answer with respect to the history of haematuria?

Answers

a. Cystectomy and urinary diversion with an ileal loop conduit which was performed for bladder carcinoma.

b. ● Hyperchloraemia
   ● Pyelonephritis
   ● Renal stones.

c. The obvious concern was that the haematuria could be due to another transitional cell carcinoma in the upper urinary tract.

Discussion

The cystectomy has been performed for transitional cell carcinoma of the bladder. An obvious concern is the possibility of another site of transitional cell carcinoma having developed in the upper urinary tract as these tumours can have multiple sites in the urothelium. Another possible cause for haematuria would have been renal calculi. To demonstrate calculi a control film is always performed as part of an IVU examination prior to contrast injection. This is because the contrast can mask calcified stones (90% of renal stones calcify). Urinary diversion into the bowel can result in complications due to reabsorption of chloride and urea leading to hyperchloraemic acidosis. Renal impairment from the recurrent pyelonephritis is also a problem. These are less of a problem with an ileal loop conduit than with a colonic urinary diversion, however. Other problems associated with urinary diversion are hypokalaemia and osteomalacia due to prolonged acidosis.

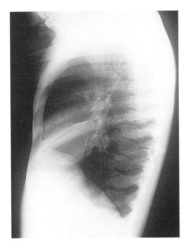 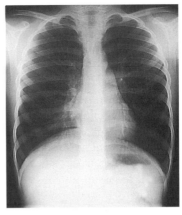

Questions

A 12-year-old boy was brought to casualty at 5 a.m. with breathlessness. On examination he looked tired and was pale. He was using the accessory muscles of respiration and his heart rate was 120 per minute and blood pressure 90/60. His chest X-ray is shown. Other investigations were as follows:

Full blood count:

- Hb 12.0 g/dl
- White cell count $11 \times 10^9/l$
- Neutrophils 60%
- Lymphocytes 20%
- Eosinophils 15%
- Basophils 2%.

Electrolytes:
- Sodium 140 mmol/l,
- Potassium 3.6 mmol/l,
- Urea 7 mmol/l.

Blood gases on air:
- pH 7.3
- pO_2 9.0 kPa
- pCO_2 5.0 kPa.

a. What is the abnormality on his chest X-ray?
b. What is the most likely cause of this?
c. What treatment should he receive?

Answers

a. Right middle lobe collapse.

b. Inspissated sputum blocking the airways in an acute asthmatic attack.

c. He is clinically very ill being hypotensive and tachycardiac. His blood gases demonstrate he is developing respiratory failure (hypoxaemia) and his differential blood count shows an eosinophilia consistent with the diagnosis of asthma. No mention is made of whether wheezes can be heard or not on auscultation of his chest. A 'silent chest' is indicative of severe asthma as the patient becomes too tired to breathe and there is severe airways obstruction. This young boy needs to be given 100% oxygen and receive intravenous fluids immediately. He should also be given intravenous hydrocortisone (200 mg) and nebulized bronchodilators (salbutamol and ipratropium bromide). Although there may be no evidence of infection, antibiotics should be given. The patient should be monitored closely, preferably on the intensive care unit, and he may need intravenous bronchodilating drugs (salbutamol, theophylline). He will need an arterial line and blood gases should be monitored every 15–30 minutes. If he does not improve ventilation should be considered. The lobar collapse will improve with this treatment and physiotherapy and rarely needs other treatment (e.g. bronchoscopy and bronchioalveolar lavage).

Discussion

When the right middle lobe becomes deaerated it collapses against the right heart border which becomes less distinct on the PA film. On the lateral film the collapsed lobe can be seen as an oblique band anteriorly in the thorax next to the heart. In a child other causes of collapse include inhalation of a foreign body (e.g. peanut) and infection and this should be borne in mind although in an asthmatic the most likely cause is inspissated sputum. In an older patient bronchial obstruction due to carcinoma should be included in the differential diagnosis. In an asthmatic it is also important to exclude on the X-ray a pneumothorax, pneumomediastinum or consolidation. The clinical signs of lobar collapse on the right side would be deviation of the trachea to the right, decreased expansion on the right with dullness to percussion and decreased air entry on auscultation.

The diagnosis of asthma is usually made on the history which is of episodic wheeze, breathlessness and cough. Wheeze is not always a feature, especially in children who may only have had a nocturnal cough for several months before they present with an acute asthmatic attack. Childhood asthma is usually associated with a family history, hay fever and eczema, whereas late onset asthma (adult asthma) is not. There are often precipitating factors (e.g. infection, exercise, cold, pollen, smoke, emotion). Despite improved treatments for asthma the incidence is increasing, as is the mortality. It is important to take all asthmatic attacks seriously although certain clinical features can be useful in judging severity:

- Dyspnoea. Inability to speak implies inability to drink and leads to dehydration and hypotension. Wheeze may be absent. The patient will be sat up using the accessory muscles of respiration
- Drowsiness and confusion This is due to hypoxaemia
- Cyanosis. Occurs at lower pO_2 than in chronic bronchitis and is a serious sign in an acute asthmatic attack
- Pulse. Tachycardia indicates the severity of an attack. Pulsus paradoxus also indicates a severe attack. Pulsus paradoxus is an exaggeration of a normal phenomenon in which there is an increased pulse pressure in expiration and a decreased pulse pressure in inspiration. This is due to the change in the intrathoracic pressure with respiration and the increase in stroke volume in expiration as the lungs squeeze blood into the heart with the resultant increase in ventricular filling. These changes in thoracic pressure are increased in an asthmatic attack and so pulsus paradoxus becomes more obvious and the pulse may be impalpable in inspiration. It is usually measured using a sphygmomanometer which makes the phenomenon more obvious and it is expressed as pulsus paradoxus demonstrated over the first 40 mmHg mercury. This gives an indication of the severity of the asthmatic attack and can be used to monitor improvement with treatment.

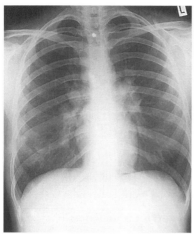

(a)

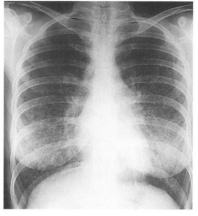

(b)

Questions

These are the chest X-rays of two patients with the same condition. One patient complained of painful lesions on her legs and breathlessness (b) and the other patient was asymptomatic (a) and had had a chest X-ray due to being in contact with a family member who had 'open' pulmonary tuberculosis.

a. Describe the abnormalities on the two radiographs.
b. What is the most likely cause of the painful lesions on her legs?
c. What is the diagnosis?

Answers

a. Bilateral hilar lymphadenopathy (BHL) is present on X-ray (b) (asymptomatic patient). The other X-ray (a) shows BHL as well as diffuse pulmonary mottling especially in the lower zones.

b. Erythema nodosum.

c. Sarcoidosis.

Discussion

The chest X-ray is usually abnormal in cases of sarcoidosis, the commonest feature being BHL but pulmonary involvement is variable:

1. **Bilateral hilar lymphadenopathy alone**. This is the commonest X-ray appearance. The glands involved are bronchopulmonary and enlarge due to the non-caseating reaction which is classical in sarcoidosis. Recovery, both radiologically and clinically, is usually complete (75% of cases).
2. **BHL and reticular-nodular (miliary) shadowing in the lung fields**. This is less common than 1 (above) but may progress to 3 (below). Clinical and radiological recovery occurs in 50% of cases.
3. **Chronic pulmonary fibrosis**. This is associated with a poor prognosis.
4. **Large nodular lung lesions**. These are uncommon but if present may be persistent for years.

Sarcoidosis is a systemic condition characterized by non-caseating granulomatosis which may affect lungs, mediastinal lymph nodes and skin. The aetiology is unknown and it mainly affects young women (20–40 years; female to male ratio = 5:1). Clinical manifestations include:

- Malaise, lassitude, generalized lymphadenopathy
- Polyarthralgia. Usually affects knees and ankles. Bone cysts can occur
- Skin: erythema nodosum, lupus pernio, sarcoid infiltration of scars
- Eyes: uveitis, keratoconjunctivitis
- Hypercalcaemia. This is due to hypersensitivity to vitamin D
- Parotitis
- Hepatosplenomegaly. Hepatic granulomas are common
- Nervous system: peripheral neuropathy, isolated cranial nerve lesions. Bilateral facial nerve palsies can occur which are sometimes difficult to diagnose due to bilateral involvement, other peripheral nerve lesions can also occur and sarcoidosis is a cause of mononeuritis multiplex.

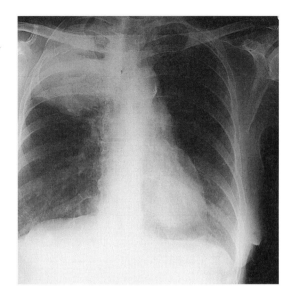

Questions

This patient complained of a 'droopy' right eyelid and pain in her shoulder. She had also become more clumsy and had been dropping objects from her right hand.

a. What is the abnormality on the chest X-ray?
b. What is the underlying diagnosis?
c. What other signs may be associated with the droopy eyelid (name three)?
d. List two reasons for her increased clumsiness.

Answers

a. There is a right upper lobe mass with cavitation. The right third rib has been destroyed.

b. Right apical bronchial carcinoma (Pancoast's tumour).

c. Miosis, enopthalmos, anhydrosis and vasodilatation all on the right side. This is Horner's syndrome.

d. Wasting of the small muscles of the hand (T1 lesion) due to local destruction by tumour, cerebellar syndrome (may occur as a non-metastatic malignant syndrome), peripheral neuropathy, cerebral secondaries, myasthenic syndrome.

Discussion

Pancoast's tumour is an apical bronchial carcinoma which causes shoulder pain by direct involvement of bone or involvement of the brachial plexus. Pressure on the C7–T1 nerve roots causes sensory and motor (wasting of the small muscles of the hand) changes. Involvement of the sympathetic chain causes Horner's syndrome. A patient may also have finger clubbing, tracheal deviation, apical lung signs and cervical lymphadenopathy. The patient may complain of other symptoms related to the bronchial carcinoma (e.g. cough, haemoptysis, fatigue, weight loss, anorexia and dyspnoea). Symptoms may be due to metastatic disease, involving bone, brain, liver, skin, kidney, etc. Bronchial carcinoma can also cause endocrine syndromes due to ectopic hormone production, e.g. ACTH, ADH, prolactin (usually from oat cell tumours) and PTH (usually from squamous cell tumours).

Other causes of Horner's syndrome are: surgery or trauma, demyelinating disease, carotid aneurysm, brain stem vascular syndromes, syringomyelia and idiopathic.

CT is the mainstay for staging of bronchogenic carcinoma, but with a Pancoast's tumour MRI can give additional information due to the ability to scan in the sagittal and coronal planes, its improved soft tissue contrast, and the ability to image the brachial plexus.

In this case, due to chest wall invasion being present, the tumour is at least stage T_3.

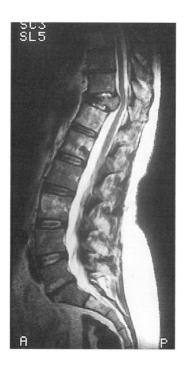

Questions

This 70-year-old lady presented with a fall. She had had a right mastectomy 10 years previously and a thyroidectomy 20 years ago but otherwise there was no past history of note. On examination she was vague but conscious. The tone was increased in her legs and power was MRC grade 2/5, reflexes were increased. There was a smooth soft mass arising from her pelvis to the level of the umbilicus. Blood tests were as follows:

- Haemoglobin 10.1 g/dl
- Potassium 5.8 mmol/l
- Sodium 154 mmol/l
- Urea 28 mmol/l

- Creatinine 140 μmol/l
- Calcium 2.7 mmol/l
- Albumin 30 g/l.

a. What is this investigation?
b. What does it show?
c. What is the most likely cause?
d. What is the mass in her pelvis?
e. What is her corrected calcium level?

Answers

a. MRI scan of lower thoracic, lumbar and sacral spine.

b. Destruction and collapse of T11 vertebral body with compression of the spinal cord at that level.

c. Bony secondaries from a primary right breast carcinoma removed 10 years previously.

d. Urinary bladder. She has signs of spinal cord compression and has developed urinary retention due to the loss of sphincter sensation which is an ominous sign. She will also have a sensory level at T11 which is not mentioned in the history. This locates the site of the lesion along with absent abnormal neurological signs above that level. There may also be lower motor neurone signs if the nerve roots are compressed by the collapsed vertebral body.

e. Corrected calcium = 2.9 mmol/l. This is corrected to an albumin of 40 g/l and the difference in the albumin is multiplied by a factor of 0.02, e.g. $(40 - 30) \times 0.02 = 0.2$; $0.2 + 2.7 = 2.9$ mmol/l. If the albumin was 50 g/l then the corrected calcium would be $2.7 - 0.2 = 2.5$ mmol/l. She is also dehydrated (hypernatraemia, uraemia and normal creatinine).

Discussion

Spinal cord compression is a neurosurgical emergency, especially if it is of recent onset and progressive. Decompression has to be performed as soon as possible if full recovery is to occur. Patients usually present with a spastic paraparesis as in this case. The sensory level indicates the site of the abnormal lesion. If there is compression of nerve roots there may be lower motor neurone signs (e.g. fasciculation, wasting), but this is more common in degenerative spine disease (e.g. cervical spondylosis). Causes of spinal cord compression can be classified as follows:

- Vertebral disorders: collapsed vertebral body (carcinoma, myeloma, osteoporosis); prolapsed intervertebral disc; canal stenosis; cervical spondylosis; abscesses; Paget's disease
- Meningeal disorders: neurofibroma; meningioma
- Spinal cord disorders: gliomas; ependymomas.

MRI scanning is now the investigation of first choice in cases of spinal cord compression. Delineation of soft tissue masses makes this investigation accurate and diagnostic. Myelography to delineate the level of the lesion is used less commonly now and it is not without risk. It remains useful, however, in those patients who cannot undergo MRI because of severe claustrophobia or some other contraindication (e.g. presence of a cardiac pacemaker, cerebral berry aneurysm clips, prosthetic cardiac valves, cochlear implants, intraocular metallic foreign bodies). The latter contraindications are relevant as MRI scanning employs a very strong magnetic field which, therefore, can affect ferromagnetic materials such as berry aneurym clips.

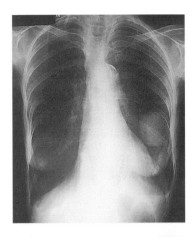

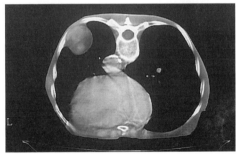

Questions

This 74-year-old lady complained of persistent back pain for 6 months. She had had a left pneumothorax at the age of 18 years. She was hypertensive and was undergoing investigations for this. She had suffered from epilepsy since she was a child.

a. What is the lesion on the images?
b. What is the diagnosis?
c. List two possible reasons for her hypertension.

Answers

a. A left intercostal neurofibroma. The smoothly rounded mass in the left mid zone on the chest X-ray can be seen to be causing pressure erosion of the rib. It is attached to the rib cage posteriorly on the CT scan image (the patient is in the prone position for CT guided biopsy).

b. Neurofibromatosis (*von Recklinghausen's disease).

c. Pheochromocytoma, renal artery stenosis. Each of these occurs in 2% of cases of neurofibromatosis.

Discussion

Neurofibromatosis is one of the most common autosomal dominant conditions affecting 20:100 000 of the population. There are two major types: peripheral and central. The peripheral type accounts for 90% of cases and its major features are: peripheral neurofibromas, café au lait spots and Lisch nodules, (pigmented iris hamartomas seen with slit lamp). Other complications include: plexiform neuromas (30%), intellectual handicap (10%), epilepsy (as in this case), sarcomatous change (6%), scoliosis (5%), spinal neurofibromas, pseudoarthrosis (3%), pheochromocytomas (2%), renal artery stenosis (2%), lung cysts (rupture of these causes pneumothoraces as in this case), rib notching. The peripheral neurofibromas cause deformity, pain and sensory disturbance. In this case there was no clinical deformity but the smooth rounded neurofibroma is attached to the inside of the rib cage and caused chronic pain. The smooth erosion of the rib with a sclerotic margin indicates a benign lesion (malignancy destroys bone that it invades). Central neurofibromatosis has few peripheral features and bilateral acoustic neuromas are the main feature. It is associated with abnormalities on chromosome 22 and there may be other 'central' features (e.g. meningioma).

---

*F.D. von Recklinghausen (1833–1910), German pathologist.

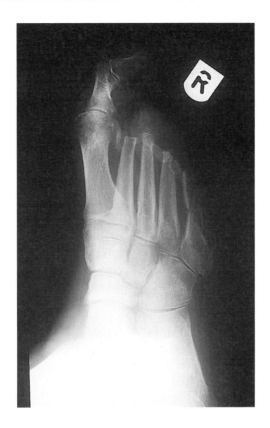

Questions

This 64-year-old man had a painless ulcer on the sole of his foot.

a. Describe the abnormalities on the X-ray (list two); what is the X-ray diagnosis?
b. What disease had caused this?

Answers

a. There is amputation of the second, third and fourth toes. There is destruction of the fifth metatarsal and the first metatarsal head secondary to osteomyelitis. The source of the infection is a neuropathic ulcer on the patient's sole.

b. Diabetes mellitus.

Discussion

Pyogenic infections of bone (with the exception of compound fractures) have become relatively rare because of the widespread use of antibiotics. Radiological changes are uncommon nowadays in the well treated case. Treatment is often delayed as the patient with a neuropathic ulcer presents late as there is no pain. There are no radiological changes in the first 2 weeks of infection then there is periosteal reaction and some osteoporosis at the site of the infection. This progresses to bony destruction, as in this case.

Osteomyelitis would normally cause severe pain, swelling and systemic upset but in a diabetic patient with peripheral neuropathy these symptoms are not always present. The commonest infecting organism is *Staphylococcus pyogenes* but other organisms (e.g. streptococcus, salmonella and *E. coli*) may be involved. The patient requires antibiotics for at least 6 weeks and may require local surgical toilet.

There are many causes of peripheral neuropathy, all of which can result in a neuropathic ulcer. The signs are sensory, motor or mixed and occur symmetrically in a 'glove and stocking' distribution. The commonest causes of the peripheral neuropathy are diabetes mellitus, alcoholism and malignancy. Causes of peripheral neuropathy can be classified as follows:

- Metabolic: diabetes mellitus; uraemia; hypothyroidism; amyloidosis.
- Malignancy: lung (this is the commonest)
- Infections: Guillain–Barré syndrome; leprosy
- Vitamin deficiency: B_{12}; B_6; thiamine and nicotinic acid deficiencies which occur mainly in alcholics
- Drugs: vincristine; vinblastine; metronidazole; isoniazid
- Inherited: perineal muscular atrophy (rare).

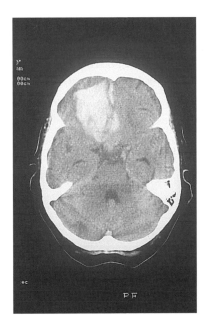 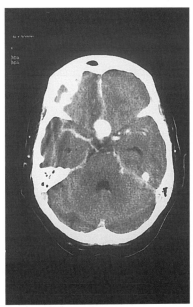

Questions

This 74-year-old lady complained of a severe headache and photophobia. On examination she was mildly confused and apyrexial. There was marked neck stiffness but no other abnormalities.

a. What two abnormalities can be seen on the two CT scan slices shown?
b. What treatment should she receive?

Answers

a. The CT scan is enhanced (vessels are seen on second scan). There is a large area of fresh blood in the right frontal area. The rounded area of the second slice is an aneurysm of the anterior communicating artery.

b. • Supportive (e.g. intravenous fluids, analgesics, oxygen)
   • Nimodipine 60 mg 4 hourly. This is to reduce the incidence of cerebral infarction
   • Neurosurgical intervention. This should be considered but the risks in this case are high.

Discussion

The most frequent cause of a subarachnoid haemorrhage in all age groups is rupture of a cerebral aneurysm. The incidence of subarachnoid haemorrhage is 15:100 000 population per year. The mortality is 50% from the initial rupture and there is a considerable morbidity. The morbidity is related to the re-bleeding that may occur as well as cerebral infarction with consequent neurological deficit. The classical presentation is the onset of a sudden severe headache which is often accompanied by vomiting, collapse and impaired consciousness. The presentation is not always classical, particularly in the elderly who may have a mild headache with neck stiffness but no other signs. There may be physical signs relating to an enlarging aneurysm, for example a posterior communicating artery aneurysm which is the commonest cause of a third cranial nerve palsy.

The first investigation of choice for a suspected subrachnoid haemorrhage is a CT scan which will reveal subarachnoid blood in 90% of cases. In the remaining 10% when a CT scan is normal a lumbar puncture is required and this should be performed at least 12 hours following the onset of the headache to allow the development of xanthochromia from red blood cell breakdown in the CSF. The combination of a CT scan and lumbar puncture will make the diagnosis in the majority of patients.

The mortality and morbidity from a subarachnoid haemorrhage is related to the initial bleed, re-bleeding and cerebral ischaemia. Management therefore should be directed to minimizing these events. Oral nimodipine 60 mg 4 hourly has shown to be well tolerated and to reduce cerebral infarction and improve outcome following the subarachnoid haemorrhage. If patients cannot take this orally then it can be given intravenously. The patient should receive supportive therapy in the form of intravenous fluid, with close monitoring of blood pressure and central venous pressure. Blood gases should be monitored and oxygen prescribed. All cases should be discussed with the neurosurgeon regarding further intervention in the form of clipping of the aneurysm. The timing of surgical intervention has been controversial. Early surgery (within 4 days) has been associated with poorer operative outcomes. However, delayed surgery is associated with an increased number of patients who succumb to re-bleeding. Age is not a contraindication to surgery. However, older patients who have previously been disabled with chronic illnesses and who have a large bleed present a high surgical risk and should be managed conservatively. The decision to intervene should be taken by the physician and neurosurgeon together and should include discussion with the family and where possible the patient.

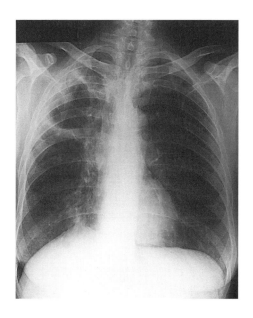

Questions

This 69-year-old lady complained of a cough, malaise and anorexia. She had had a flu-like illness 2 weeks previously. On examination she looked ill and had a temperature of 39.5°C. Her blood pressure was 90/60 and pulse 120 per minute. Her blood results were as follows:

- Haemoglobin 11.1 g/dl
- White cell count $32 \times 10^9/l$
- Sodium 120 mmol/l
- Potassium 3.8 mmol/l
- Urea 18 mmol/l
- ESR 78 mm/hr.

a. What is the abnormality on the chest X-ray?
b. What is the most likely cause of this abnormality?
c. What is the most likely cause of her hyponatraemia?
d. What treatment should she receive?

Answers

a. There is a large cystic lesion which contains a fluid level in the right upper lobe. It is a lung abscess.

b. It is most likely due to a staphylococcal pneumonia following on from influenza. There are, however, several causes of lung abscesses (see below).

c. Inappropriate ADH secretion.

d. Following blood and sputum cultures she should receive intravenous normal saline and intravenous flucloxacillin. Her blood gases should be monitored as should her fluid balance and vital signs. Supportive therapy including postural drainage and physiotherapy is usually all that is required. Surgical excision is rarely required.

Discussion

Causes of lung abscesses can be classified as follows:

- Bronchial obstruction (by a carcinoma or foreign body)
- Aspiration
- Following or an association with pneumonia particularly staphylococcus, klebsiella and pneumococcus. It can also occur in association with tubercle and actinomyces
- Vascular emboli (e.g. pulmonary infarct or emboli from a pyaemia)
- Infected congenital or acquired cyst.

Clinically there is usually systemic upset and the patient is very ill with a swinging fever. There is often purulent sputum which is foul smelling and the white cell count is high. If an underlying obstructing lesion is thought likely bronchoscopy must be performed. Management as above with intravenous fluids and antibiotics is required.

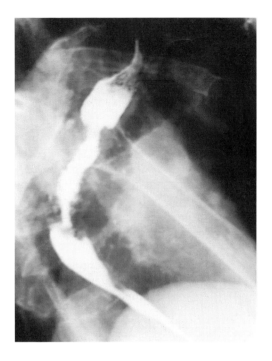

Questions

This patient complained of nausea, anorexia and chest pain.

a. What is this investigation?
b. What is the diagnosis?

Answers

a. Barium swallow.

b. Carcinoma of the middle third of the oesophagus.

Discussion

There is an irregular, long ('apple core') structure of the middle third of the oesophagus. Carcinomas of the oesophagus can occur in the upper, middle or lower third. There is usually little diagnostic difficulty on a barium meal as benign strictures tend to be smooth but oesophagoscopy and biospy should be performed to confirm the diagnosis histologically. Oesophagoscopy with dilatation is therapeutic in most cases as dysphagia is one of the most distressing symptoms patients present with. Treatment is usually palliative as presentation is often late. Some cases are suitable for surgery and radiotherapy provided there is no evidence of spread. Other palliative measures apart from dilatation include the insertion of oesophageal tubes (Celesten) and, more recently, expandable stents to relieve symptoms.

Oesophageal carcinoma is commoner in men (3:1) and in the Japanese population. Histology is usually squamous cell except in the lower third when it may be an adenocarcinoma. Lower third carcinomas are commoner in women. Symptoms include: dysphagia, nausea, anorexia, vomiting, weight loss and fatigue. Rarely perforation can occur spontaneously and is usually terminal but is more likely to occur in association with instrumentation and dilatation. Overall survival is poor (10% at 5 years).

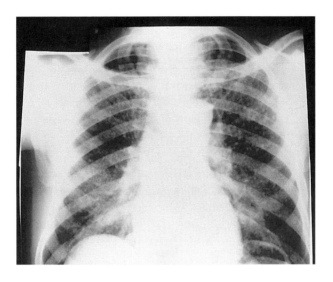

Questions

This 78-year-old vagrant was brought to casualty by a policeman who found him on the street. He was drowsy but responded to commands and was unkempt. His temperature was 38°C and there were bilateral basal crackles on auscultation of his chest. He had tar staining of his fingers and an old paramedian abdominal incision. His spleen was just palpable. Examination of his legs revealed increased tone and hyperreflexia on both sides. His blood tests revealed the following:

- Haemoglobin 9.6 g/dl
- White cell count $2.4 \times 10^9/l$
- Platelets $186 \times 10^9/l$
- MCV 100 fl
- Sodium 128 mmol/l
- Urea 21 mmol/l
- Bilirubin 55 µmol/l
- Alkaline phosphatase 206 IU/l
- Aspartate aminotransferase 88 IU/l.

a. What is the most likely cause of his chest X-ray appearance?
b. What are the possible causes (name two) of his drowsiness?
c. What is the most likely explanation for his blood results?
d. What is the probable cause of his paramedian abdominal scar?

Answers

a. Miliary mottling secondary to miliary tuberculosis.

b. Tuberculous meningitis, subdural haematoma (he was found on the street and had probably fallen). It is unlikely that he is drowsy due to hyponatraemia. He requires a CT scan of his head to exclude an intracerebral bleed, particularly in view of the neurological signs in his legs.

c. He has a megaloblastic anaemia which could be due to B_{12} and/or folate deficiency (low white cell count, low platelet count and macrocytosis points to a megaloblastic anaemia). His splenomegaly may be due to megaloblastic anaemia and the pyramidal signs in his legs could represent subacute combined degeneration of the cord due to B_{12} deficiency. The hyponatraemia is probably secondary to inappropriate ADH secretion due to miliary tuberculosis. His abnormal liver function tests may be due to miliary tuberculosis or an excess alcohol intake. The latter may also cause a macrocytosis. It is important to note that he had tar staining of his fingers and therefore is a smoker and all these features could be related to a metastatic bronchial carcinoma.

d. He probably has had a partial gastrectomy for a peptic ulcer which has predisposed him to both tuberculosis and B_{12} deficiency.

Discussion

There are many causes of nodular shadowing on a chest X-ray: tuberculosis, sarcoidosis, viral pneumonia, pneumoconiosis, rheumatoid arthritis, fungal infection, metastases and drugs (e.g. busulphan). With this clinical picture miliary tuberculosis is the most likely. The incidence of tuberculosis is increasing. Certain factors increase predisposition to infection with tubercle, e.g. ageing (due to decreased cell mediated immunity), alcoholism, vagrant lifestyle, previous partial gastrectomy. This patient fulfilled all these categories. Miliary tuberculosis is also known as 'disseminated', 'cryptic' or 'concealed' tuberculosis. The diagnosis is often difficult to make in old age, hence the last two terms. The chest X-ray is only abnormal in 50% of cases. Unfortunately the diagnosis is often made at postmortem.

Symptoms are often non-specific: weight loss, anorexia. There is often hyponatraemia due to inappropriate ADH secretion and abnormal liver function tests (especially a raised alkaline phosphatase). There may be a pancytopenia because of bone marrow suppression, as in this case, and bone marrow biopsy and culture often grows tuberculous bacilli and this can be of help in diagnosis. This patient may have both the megaloblastic anaemia and tubercle infiltration of the marrow and a bone marrow biopsy is needed to make the diagnosis. Hepatosplenomegaly is common and choroidal tubercles should be looked for on ophthalmoscopy. Quadruple anti-tuberculous therapy is needed for 6 months. This is because there is an increasing number of resistant organisms. Oral steroids are sometimes useful in conjunction with anti-tuberculous drugs to reduce inflammation and improve well-being but their use should be closely monitored.

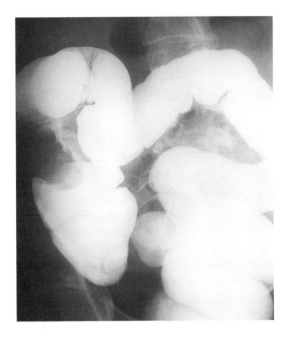

Questions

This 58-year-old woman complained of constipation and intermittent abdominal pain. She was tired and also had had dyspnoea on exertion and palpitations for 2 months.

a. What is this investigation?
b. What does it show?
c. What is the most likely cause of her cardiovascular symptoms?
d. What is the treatment?

Answers

a. Barium enema (single contrast in this case).

b. Carcinoma of the ascending colon ('apple core' lesion).

c. Iron deficiency anaemia.

d. Right hemicolectomy.

Discussion

The symptoms and signs at presentation of a colonic carcinoma are determined by its stage. This patient clearly had had anaemia due to occult blood loss for several weeks. Iron deficiency anaemia is a common presentation particularly of caecal carcinoma in the elderly. All cases of iron deficiency should be fully investigated and a cause found. Altered bowel habit is a common symptom. Symptoms of intestinal obstruction (colicky abdominal pain, nausea, vomiting, abdominal distension and constipation) may develop as the bowel lumen becomes occluded. The treatment almost always includes surgery for both curative and palliative reasons but the indications for chemotherapy accompanying surgery depend upon the stage of the carcinoma.

The barium enema remains the mainstay of investigation with colonoscopy needed for biopsy when a suspicious area is found. Here, however, there is no doubt. Ultrasound is useful to exclude liver metastases. CT or MRI is used to stage some cases, especially rectal and anal tumours.

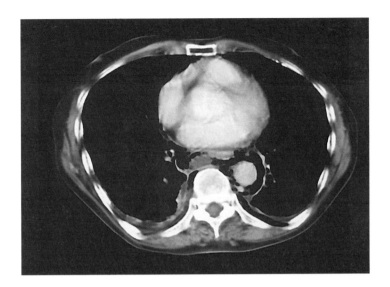

Questions

This patient had just returned from the theatre after a procedure. He complained of pain in his chest and neck and on examination looked ill with a heart rate of 120 per minute and blood pressure 100/70.

a. What can be seen on this CT scan?
b. What procedure has he just had to cause this appearance?
c. What physical sign confirming the diagnosis may be present?

Answers

a. This is a CT scan of his thorax showing air in the mediastinum (black) which surrounds the mediastinal structures and there is a pneumothorax on the right side (can be seen posteriorly).

b. Oesophageal dilatation resulting in a perforated oesophagus.

c. Surgical emphysema may be present as air tracks upwards through the soft tissues and most commonly is felt as 'crackling' swellings in the supraclavicular fossa.

Discussion

Causes of oesophageal perforation are:

- Iatrogenic. Following oesophageal dilatation for peptic strictures or carcinoma and following biopsy
- Foreign bodies (e.g. fish bone)
- Perforating wounds
- Spontaneous. Usually lower thoracic and this is uncommon. It may follow prolonged retching.

The patient complains of pain in the chest, neck and upper abdomen. The patient is usually ill and may be pyrexial and shocked. Surgical or subcutaneous emphysema points to the diagnosis. There may be a 'click' which is a rhythmical sound heard on auscultation of the heart and occurs when a small left pneumothorax is present between the layers of the mediastinal pleura. Cardiac systole has a sharp impact between the layers of pleura producing the click which is similar to the sound produced by snapping the fingers. Surgical emphysema can be confirmed by a chest X-ray which may also show a pneumomediastinum, pneumothorax or hydrothorax. A water-soluble contrast swallow will confirm the perforation and its position. If perforation is in the cervical region it is managed conservatively, keeping the patient nil by mouth and giving intravenous fluids and antibiotics. Other perforations usually require surgical intervention. There is a high mortality.

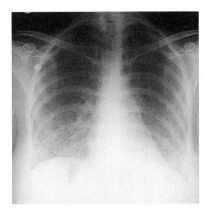

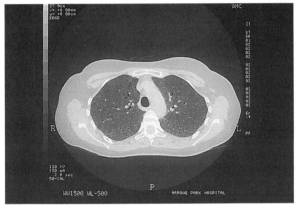

Questions

This patient complained of a dry cough for 6 months and recurrent episodes of dyspnoea. She was on no medication and was a non-smoker. She lived alone and had a parrot, dog and a cat.

a. What are the abnormalities (name one) on each film?
b. What other symptoms may she have (list three)?
c. What is the diagnosis?

Answers

a. Diffuse shadowing on the chest X-ray and the high resolution CT scan of the thorax shows diffuse nodularity and ground glass shadowing.

b. Fever, malaise, anorexia, myalgia, arthralgia. Symptoms due to cor pulmonale (ankle oedema) may occur and this is a late feature.

c. Extrinsic allergic alveolitis (probably caused by the parrot; bird-fancier's lung).

Discussion

Extrinsic allergic alveolitis is produced by a type III allergic reaction in the alveoli and bronchioles to organic dusts. Precipitins can be demonstrated, usually in the serum. There are several types of extrinsic allergic alveolitis depending upon the antigen involved; the most commonly known is farmer's lung which is triggered by mouldy hay. Other examples include: mushroom worker's lung (spores of actinomycetes in mould); bird-fancier's lung (avian antigens from feathers, excreta, etc.); malt workers lung (spores of *Aspergillus clavatus*).

Pathologically the alveolar walls become thickened and there is infiltration of lymphocytes, plasma cells and polymorphs. Advanced cases develop granulomata and diffuse lung fibrosis. The patient develops the symptoms usually after exposure to the antigen. It takes about 4–6 hours for the symptoms to develop, and they subside in about 2–3 days. After acute attacks pulmonary fibrosis may develop. On examination there may be finger clubbing if pulmonary fibrosis has developed. Lung expansion will be limited and there will be fine, late inspiratory crackles at the bases of the lungs. Pulmonary function tests will show a restrictive picture with a low transfer factor during acute attacks and in the chronic phase. Blood gases show a reduced pO_2 and the pCO_2 is normal or reduced (type I respiratory failure). The chest X-ray can show diffuse hazy shadowing, nodularity, as in this case, or frank pulmonary fibrosis (especially upper lobes). The appearance may represent a mixture of all three types of shadowing. It partially depends on the pattern of exposure: a large sudden exposure (such as the farmer working with hay), or a chronic, low level, constant exposure (such as from a bird cage). The latter may have progressed to fibrosis by the time of presentation.

Treatment includes avoiding the responsible antigen which is the most important measure. Steroid therapy is useful in the first attacks in the acute phase but steroids are of little use once pulmonary fibrosis has developed. Other treatments are supportive (e.g. oxygen therapy).

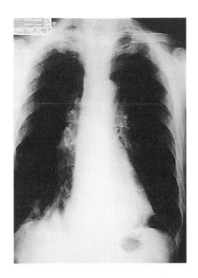

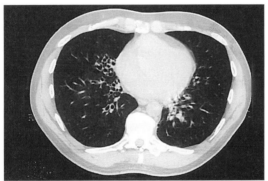

Questions

These images belong to two patients with the same pulmonary pathology. One patient, as well as respiratory symptoms, also has chronic oedema of the legs and brittle dystrophic nails.

a. What is the respiratory diagnosis?
b. What symptoms (list three) may the patients have?
c. What is the associated diagnosis in one patient?

Answers

a. Bronchiectasis. The chest X-ray shows hyperinflated lung fields and tubular, mucous filled bronchi at the right base. The CT scan shows 'cystic changes' extensively throughout the lungs (ectatic bronchi in this case) with thickening of the dilated airways implying chronicity.

b. Dyspnoea, wheeze, cough productive of copious sputum, haemoptysis. Intermittent infective episodes occur which produce worsening of the symptoms with more copious sputum and pleuritic chest pain. In the chronic stages of the disease cor pulmonale also develops producing ankle oedema.

c. Yellow nail syndrome.

Discussion

Bronchiectasis means dilatation of the distal airways. There are several causes of this, as follows:

- Infections (measles, whooping cough, pneumonia)
- Obstructive lesions (foreign bodies, such as peanuts, and bronchial carcinoma)
- Pulmonary tuberculosis (this is less common than previously)
- Cystic fibrosis
- Congenital (Kartagener's syndrome: situs inversus, sinusitus, bronchiectasis)
- Yellow nail syndrome.

The patient with bronchiectasis usually has a chronic cough which is often postural and which classically produces copious amounts of sputum (several cupfuls a day). This is exacerbated by acute infections. The patient has halitosis due to this. There may be haemoptysis due to destruction of the bronchial veins and this can sometimes be quite severe. There is dyspnoea and wheeze and in advanced cases cachexia and cor pulmonale. The patient becomes a respiratory cripple (in cases of cystic fibrosis) and respiratory failure is the terminal event. On examination there is finger clubbing (due to chronic pulmonary sepsis) and central cyanosis. There will be extensive wheezes and crackles on auscultation of the lung fields and there may be associated lobar collapse and pleural effusions. Cerebral abscess is a recognized complication if pyogenic emboli occur.

Treatment includes physiotherapy which is daily with postural drainage to empty the dilated airways and reduce the incidence of further infective episodes. Other supportive therapy (e.g. oxygen, bron-chodilators, steroids and antibiotics) are used as necessary.

Yellow nail syndrome consists of: yellow nails which are brittle and dys-trophic and may shed and re-grow, bronchiectasis, sinusitis, chylous pleural effusions, chylous ascites and lymphoedema. The pathological abnormality is lymphangectasia. Cases are sporadic and are commoner in females over the age of 50 years.

High resolution CT has replaced bronchography as the investigation of choice for suspected bronchiectasis. Diagnosis on a plain chest radio-graph is rarely as easy as in the case shown here.

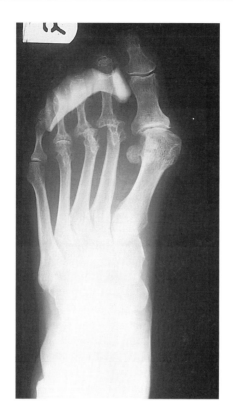

Questions

This patient had sudden onset of foot drop and an X-ray of her foot was requested.

a. What does it show (list three abnormalities)?
b. What is the diagnosis?
c. What is the probable cause of her foot drop?

Answers

a. Subluxation of the metatarsophalangeal joints with narrowing of the joint spaces, periarticular osteoporosis and erosions.

b. Rheumatoid arthritis.

c. Mononeuritis multiplex involving the lateral popliteal nerve.

Discussion

Rheumatoid arthritis is more commonly seen in women (3:1) and there is often a family history. It is a multi-system disorder. The arthritis typically involves the small joints of the hands and feet, most commonly in a symmetrical fashion but large synovial joints (e.g. knees, elbows) are often involved. The onset is insidious with morning stiffness and swelling of joints. Characteristically the metacarpophalangeal joints are swollen with ulnar deviation. The proximal interphalangeal joints may be involved but the distal interphalangeal joints are spared. Similarly the metatarsophalangeal joints may be involved. There is often wasting of the small muscles of the hands. Rheumatoid arthritis is a cause of mononeuritis multiplex as in this case. Other causes of mononeuritis multiplex include diabetes mellitus, multiple sclerosis, Wegener's granulomatosis and sarcoidosis. The onset of mononeuritis multiplex is typically sudden due to involvement of the vascular supply to the nerve. Other neurological associations of rheumatoid arthritis include peripheral neuropathy, carpal tunnel syndrome, cord lesions due to cervical disease and lesions due to atlantoaxial subluxation. Other systems involved in rheumatoid disease include:

- Respiratory: pleural effusion, rheumatoid nodules, fibrosing alveolitis, Caplan's syndrome
- Cardiovascular: pericarditis, splinter haemorrhages, nail fold infarcts, vasculitis of the skin, leg ulcers, Raynaud's phenomenon
- Haematological: normochromic/normocytic anaemia, splenomegaly (5% of cases), leucopenia (1% of cases), generalized lymphadenopathy (10% of cases)
- Kidneys: amyloidosis may occur secondary to this chronic inflammatory condition
- Eyes: keratoconjunctivitis, scleritis, scleromalacia perforans.

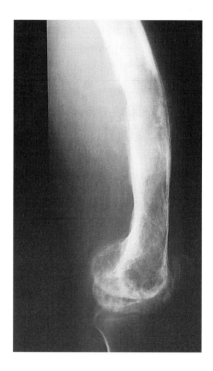

Questions

This 78-year-old man complained of pain in his leg. He had lost 2 stones in weight over the last 3 months and had developed polyuria and poly-dipsia. Routine urine testing was normal. He was deaf.

a. What does the X-ray show?
b. What complication has developed?
c. What is the most likely reason for his polyuria and polydipsia?
d. List two reasons for his deafness.

Answers

a. The shaft of the femur shows extensive disorganization of bone with thickening and bowing deformity. This is Paget's disease of bone.

b. Sarcomatous change. There is loss of the cortex posteriorly with erosive/lytic changes.

c. He most likely has hypercalcaemia which has been exacerbated by his immobility secondary to pain. He has the classical symptoms of diabetes mellitus (polyuria, polydipsia and weight loss) but it is mentioned that his urine testing was negative.

d. Compression of the auditory nerve in the auditory canal due to enlargement of the skull by Paget's disease. Involvement of the ear ossicles in the pagetic process.

Discussion

Paget's disease of bone affects 1% of the population over the age of 50 years and is more common in men. There is a familial association. It is characterized by increased bone resorption and abnormal new bone formation. It is clinically significant in only about 10% of cases and in the remainder it is discovered incidentally on X-rays or there is an elevated serum alkaline phosphatase.

The axial skeleton (skull, pelvis) is most commonly involved in the Pagetic process followed by the limb bones. The patient may complain of bone pain and tenderness and there may be a rise in temperature over the area involved. There is often deformity (e.g. enlargement of the skull and bowing of the legs). Complications of Paget's disease include:

- Pathological fracture (this leads to hypercalcaemia and hypercalciuria, particularly when the patient is immobilized)
- Sarcomatous change (1% of cases), especially by osteogenic sarcoma, fibrosarcoma and chondrosarcoma
- Occlusion of skull foramina may cause deafness and neurological signs due to basilar invagination. Spinal stenosis is more common
- High output cardiac failure (rare).

The disease can be monitored by measuring the serum alkaline phosphatase and the 24 hour urinary hydroxyproline level. These parameters reflect the severity of the disease. Treatment is symptomatic (analgesics); other drugs which reduce the disease activity (e.g. biphosphonates, calcitonin and also mithramycin) have also been used

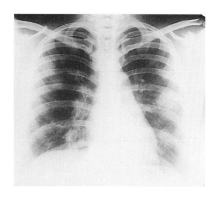 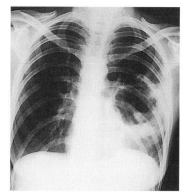

Questions

This 40-year-old woman complained of a persistent dry cough and breathlessness. She had been treated with antibiotics by her general practitioner for an episode of sinusitis 2 months previously. She complained of a painful knee and ankle and general malaise. On examination she had evidence of a peripheral neuropathy and a swollen right knee and ankle. She looked pale. Her blood results were as follows: Hb 10.1 g/dl, white cell count 12.0×10^9/l, ESR 88 mm/hr, urea 23 mmol/l, creatinine 400 µmol/l. The second chest radiograph belongs to a different patient with the same disease process.

a. What abnormalities are seen on the two chest X-rays?
b. What is the diagnosis?
c. What two investigations would most help you confirm this diagnosis?

Answers

a. There are peripheral soft opacities in both mid and lower zones on one of the films. The other chest X-ray shows a large cystic lesion which has developed in the left mid zone.

b. *Wegener's granulomatosis.

c. cANCA, transbronchial biopsy at bronchoscopy or biopsy of the nasal cavity if abnormal would be helpful to confirm the histological diagnosis.

Discussion

Wegener's granulomatosis is a granulomatous, necrotizing vasculitis involving the upper and lower respiratory tract producing epistaxis, sinusitis and destruction of the nasal cartilage (saddle nose). There can be pulmonary nodules and diffuse infiltrates which may be fleeting or which may become cystic as in this case. Respiratory symptoms develop (e.g. cough, chest pain, dyspnoea and haemoptysis). This condition is a multi-system disorder and the next most common organ involved is the kidney where there is a glomerulonephritis and renal failure can develop. The frequency of involvement of systems is as follows: respiratory tract (92%), kidney (85%), musculoskeletal system (67%), eye (52%), skin (46%), peripheral nervous system (15%), central nervous system (8%). The patient most commonly presents with fever, malaise, respiratory symptoms and a migratory arthritis as in this case. The disease affects females and males equally and most commonly presents in adulthood.

There is a vasculitis of the capillaries which results in thrombosis and occlusion of the blood vessel lumen which in turn leads to necrosis. This necrotizing vasculitis and granulomatous infiltration are the histological hallmarks of this disease. The granulomatous formation may mimic mycobacterial and fungal infection which need to be excluded as part of the differential diagnosis.

The serum contains antibodies reacting with the cytoplasm of human neutrophils (cANCA) in 90% of patients with Wegener's granulomatosis. Perinuclear ANCA (pANCA) are found in patients with cresentic glomerulonephritis whether or not in association with Wegener's granulomatosis so cANCA is more sensitive for Wegener's granulomatosis. However, in the absence of renal disease in Wegener's granulomatosis the sensitivity of cANCA is reduced to 70% of cases. False positives occur in infective and neoplastic disorders and therefore it is essential to have a histological diagnosis.

Untreated Wegener's granulomatosis has a mean survival of 5 months. Treatment with combination of oral prednisolone and low dose daily cyclophosphamide improves survival. However, cyclophosphamide is associated with serious long term toxic effects (bladder carcinoma, sterility, cystitis, myelodysplasia). In view of the possibility of sterility females are offered egg sequestration and males sperm storage before treatment with cyclophosphamide. Monthly high dose cyclophosphamide is less effective than low dose daily regimes but less toxic. Other therapies (azathioprine and cyclosporine) have been shown to be less effective. Isolated sinus disease can be treated with saline irrigation. Arthralgia and arthritis are treated symptomatically with non-steroidal anti-inflammatory drugs.

---

*F. Wegener (1907–1990), German pathologist.

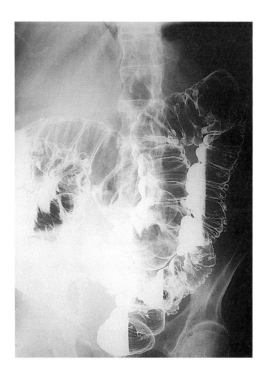

Questions

This 80-year-old man complained of intermittent diarrhoea for 6 weeks.

a. What investigation is shown?
b. List two abnormalities.
c. What is the underlying diagnosis?
d. What other symptoms (list three) may he have?

Answers

a. Double contrast barium enema.

b. There are scattered diverticula in the colon. The spinal ligaments are calcified ('bamboo spine'). The sacroiliac joints are narrow and irregular (sacroileitis).

c. Ankylosing spondylitis.

d. Backache, restricted spinal movement, morning stiffness, dyspnoea due to restricted rib cage movement. (He may have several other symptoms related to the disease (see below) but the answer should be specific to the slides shown which will gain more marks.)

Discussion

Ankylosing spondylitis is more common in men (9:1) and the onset is usually in the 3rd decade. There is a familial incidence and there is an association with HLA B27 which is present in 90% of cases. Other diseases which have a higher incidence of HLA B27 than in the general population and therefore are associated with ankylosing spondylitis are as follows: psoriasis, *Reiter's disease, inflammatory bowel disease, *Behçet's disease. Behçet's syndrome, however, is more likely to have HLA B5 associated with it. Patients with ankylosing spondylitis therefore are more likely to have an associated colitis this could have been the reason for this gentleman's diarrhoea but his barium enema did not show any evidence of this. He may have psoriasis which should be sought on examination.

During the early stages of this condition the sacroiliac joints are often affected (sacroiliitis), causing low back pain and morning stiffness. The disease then goes on to involve the whole spine producing pain, stiffness and restricted movement. The spinal ligaments become calcified and eventually ossify. The hips are involved in 50% of patients and other large joints (e.g. knees and ankles) are usually involved. A minority of cases (15%) present with a peripheral arthropathy. The arthropathy is asymmetrical and is distinguished from rheumatoid arthritis. Rheumatoid factor is negative. Other complications include:

- Anterior uveitis (40% of cases)
- Pulmonary fibrosis (1% of cases usually apical). Respiratory failure may occur due to this as well as restricted thoracic movement due to a fused spine. There is a restrictive respiratory picture

- Aortic regurgitation (1% of cases)
- Other associations (e.g. colitis, psoriasis, etc.).

The disease is progressive and is managed essentially symptomatically. Bed rest should be avoided as this increases stiffness and ankylosis. Spinal exercises are essential to avoid deformity. Non-steroidal anti-inflammatory drugs are used for analgesic purposes. Radiotherapy is effective in reducing pain but there is an increased risk of leukaemia. In severe cases ankylosis of the spine with disability and impaired ventilation occurs within 3–5 years but most cases (70%) maintain complete independence for many more years with physiotherapy and expert treatment.

*H.G. Reiter (1881–1969), German bacteriologist.
*H. Behçet (1889–1948), Turkish dermatologist.

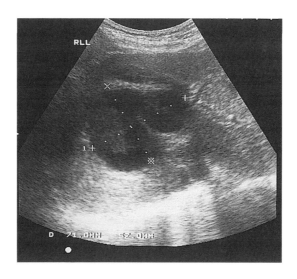

Questions

This 69-year-old lady had just returned home after visiting her daughter in the Middle East. She complained of nausea, vomiting and rigors for 3 days. On examination her temperature was 39.5°C and her heart rate was 100 per minute. Blood pressure was 120/80. She had right upper quadrant tenderness and guarding and her bowel sounds were normal.

a. What is this investigation?
b. What is the diagnosis?
c. What may her chest X-ray show (list three abnormalities)?
d. How would you confirm the diagnosis?
e. What is the treatment?

Answers

a. Liver ultrasound scan.

b. There is a single cavity containing fluid and septa. It is an abscess cavity and in view of the history above with travel to the Middle East an amoebic liver abscess is the most likely diagnosis.

c. Abscesses enlarge upwards and the chest X-ray may therefore show an elevated right hemidiaphragm, basal shadowing, basal atelectasis or a small right pleural effusion.

d. A serum antibody test for *Entamoeba histolytica* is positive in 90% of cases. Amoebae are seldom found in the faeces. The abscess can be aspirated and organisms identified but this is rarely necessary.

e. Metronidazole 400 mg tds for 7 days is required. This may have to be repeated. Surgical drainage is rarely required. When prescribing metronidazole patients should be told to avoid alcohol as there is an antabuse type reaction but the patient would be best avoiding alcohol in this case anyhow. Prolonged use of metronidazole also can result in a peripheral neuropathy. Other side-effects include nausea, vomiting, rashes, headaches, dizziness, ataxia, darkening of the urine, and leukopenia. Other treatment such as emetine and chloroquine are less effective and more toxic.

Discussion

Amoebic liver abscesses can occur without any preceding dysenteric illness. The disease is caused by the protozoal organism *Entamoeba histolytica*. The disease is endemic in Asia, Africa, the Middle East and South and Central America. The disease spreads via the faecal–oral route and is contracted from infected food or drinking water. Hepatic amoebiasis presents with a persistent fever, systemic upset and upper abdominal pain. The liver is enlarged and tender. Other causes of liver abscesses are as follows:

- Portal pyaemia from intra-abdominal sepsis, particularly acute appendicits and diverticulitis
- Actinomycosis. This is spread to the liver via the portal blood stream from the ileocaecal actinomycosis

- Biliary infection. Multiple liver abscesses may form in association with a suppurative cholangitis secondary to impacted gall stones in the common bile duct.

The clinical presentation of liver abscess, whatever the cause, is the same, with considerable systemic upset, and if not treated promptly and effectively the morbidity and mortality is substantial.

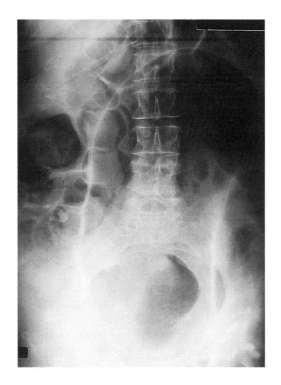

Questions

This plain abdominal film belongs to an 80-year-old man.

a. List three symptoms he may have.
b. What is the diagnosis?
c. What is the treatment?

Answers

a. Colicky abdominal pain, abdominal distension, vomiting, constipation.

b. Sigmoid volvulus. The sigmoid can be seen extemely dilated on the left side of the film.

c. A rectal tube passed through a sigmoidoscope often deflates the volvulus in the early stages. This is accompanied by passage of a large amount of flatus. If this fails the volvulus has to be untwisted at laparotomy.

Discussion

A sigmoid volvulus is more common in the elderly and more common in men (4:1). It is precipitated by constipation and is relatively uncommon in Britain, being more common in Russia, Scandinavia and among Africans. As well as constipation precipitating the event, patients with a particularly long sigmoid loop are more predisposed. The loop of sigmoid colon twists anticlockwise from a half to three turns. The clinical features are of acute intestinal obstruction and if left untreated the bowel becomes gangrenous resulting in peritonitis and death. If the passage of a flatus tube is unsuccessful then a laparotomy is required and often resection of the redundant sigmoid loop is necessary to prevent the recurrent volvulus. If gangrene has already occurred then the segment affected has to be excised and a temporary colostomy is fashioned which will later be closed.

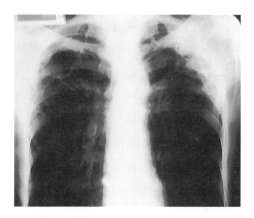

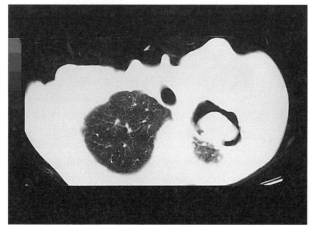

Questions

These images are from two patients who both complained of haemoptysis.

a. What is the diagnosis?
b. How would you confirm it?
c. What is the treatment?

Answers

a. There is an aspergilloma (mycetoma) in the left apex. The chest X-ray shows increased opacity in the left apex; there is often a 'halo' of air that can be seen around this which is just visible on this film. This is encircling the fungal ball which occupies the cavity (usually an old TB cavity or fibrocystic disease). There is also a large bulla in the right apex and bilateral upper lobe fibrosis on this chest radiograph. The aspergilloma is more obvious on the second patient's CT scan.

b. Aspergillus precipitins in the serum are usually positive.

c. Patients are often asymptomatic and therefore no treatment is required. Haemoptysis is the commonest problem and it may be massive. Surgical resection is required for haemoptysis, providing respiratory reserve is adequate.

Discussion

A mycetoma or aspergilloma is formed following infection with the mould *Aspergillus fumigatus*. The fungal ball usually develops in cavities which have been formed due to old tuberculous infection or cystic disease. The mycetomas have a classical X-ray appearance as described above. They enlarge very slowly and the main symptom they produce is haemoptysis. A mycetoma is only one presentation of the pulmonary effects of *A. fumigatus*; others are allergic bronchopulmonary aspergillosis or invasive aspergillosis. In all cases there is alteration or impairment of the immune reaction. In the case of a mycetoma the cavity is a safe haven for the fungus. A broad spectrum of disease is therefore produced by this agent, ranging from asymptomatic through allergic aspergillosis, causing asthma and fleeting lung shadows as well as pulmonary eosinophilia, to a mycetoma and an invasive form of aspergillosis when there is generalized systemic infection by aspergillus; this last is usually seen in immunocompromised patients and is the only one in which antifungal treatment is important and effective. The drug of choice is intravenous amphotericin B. Ketoconazole is an alternative treatment.

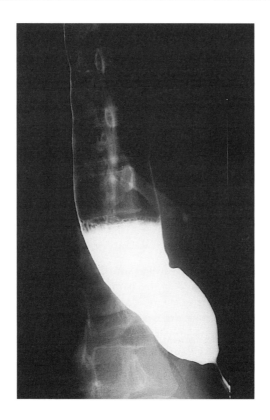

Questions

a. What is this investigation?
b. What is the diagnosis?
c. List three symptoms the patient may have.
d. List three possible treatments.

Answers

a. Barium swallow.

b. Achalasia. The 'beak-like' narrowing at the lower end of the oesphagus with massive dilatation above it is characteristic of this motility disorder which is due to failure of relaxation of the lower oesophageal sphincter.

c. Dysphagia, chest pain, regurgitation/vomiting and symptoms due to aspiration pneumonia which is common.

d. Endoscopic dilatation (often needs repeating at intervals), cardiomyotomy, (Heller's operation), endoscopic injection of botulinum toxin.

Discussion

Achalasia of the cardia or cardiospasm is a neuromuscular failure of relaxation of the lower end of the oesophagus. This causes progressive dilatation and tortuosity of the oesophagus with incoordination of peristalsis and hypertrophy of the oesophagus above the lesion. It typically presents after the age of 30 years and is more common in females (3:2). The main symptoms are dysphagia and regurgitation of food which cannot pass through the lower end of the oesophagus. Recurrent episodes of pneumonia due to aspiration may be the presenting feature. The chest X-ray, as well as showing evidence of aspiration pneumonia, may reveal a mediastinal mass produced by the dilated oesophagus. A barium swallow confirms the diagnosis which has a typical appearance as in this case.

The mainstay of treatment of this condition is endoscopic dilatation. More recently injection of botulinum toxin into the lower oesophageal sphincter at endoscopy has been shown in clinical trials to improve symptoms of dysphagia, chest pain and regurgitation in up to 90% of patients. 80–100 units are injected into the lower oesophageal sphincter. Repeated injections are necessary for a therapeutic effect. Botulinum toxin reduces lower oesophageal sphincter tone. Some patients have benefited for up to 2 years following one injection and older patients (over the age of 50 years) have a better response than younger patients. This can be a useful treatment as repeated oesophageal dilatation carries a risk of perforation. Surgery should be used as a last resort.

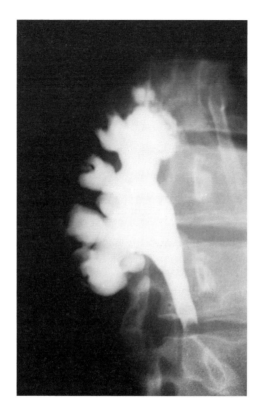

Questions

This patient has had rheumatoid arthritis for 30 years.

a. What is this investigation?
b. What is the diagnosis?
c. List three other causes of this condition.

Answers

a. An intravenous urogram.

b. Papillary necrosis due to analgesic nephropathy.

c. Obstructive uropathy, renal tuberculosis, acute pyelonephritis (especially in diabetics), sickle cell disease, alcoholism.

Discussion

Papillary necrosis is usually due to ischaemia caused by damage to the medullary blood supply. Then papillae become eroded and clubbed. The picture may be complicated by repeated urinary tract infections, renal stone formation or an obstructive uropathy. In the case of analgesic nephropathy due to phenacetin the papillary necrosis may be due to direct toxicity from the drug and these patients are predisposed to carcinoma of the renal pelvis.

Symptoms of renal failure are often non-specific (e.g. anorexia, malaise). There may be urinary symptoms (e.g. polyuria, oliguria). Itching is a common symptom. It is important to take a full history including drug history and family history (hypertension, polycystic kidney disease and gout). Clinical signs associated with renal failure include a brownish pallor of uraemic anaemia and there may be a brown line near the end of the finger nails. Bruising is more common and the patient may be hyperventilating due to acidosis. The patient may be dehydrated (dry, non-elastic skin and sunken eyes) or have fluid retention (ankle oedema, signs of congestive heart failure). There may be evidence of a peripheral neuropathy. In the end stages of renal failure there may be pericarditis, muscular twitching, hiccough, and uraemic frost. This is crystals of urea which are white and can be seen on the skin especially around the eyes and nose.

Radiologically, in the early stages there is swelling of the papillae. Later partial or total sloughing or necrosis in situ occurs. The calyces appear dilated when the papillae have been sloughed. The papillae themselves can cause obstruction like calculi and can calcify. Both partial and total sloughing of papillae is seen in this case.

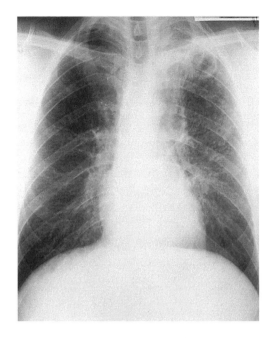

Questions

This is the chest X-ray of a 78-year-old man who complained of a persistent cough for 6 months. He was on long term steroids for temporal arteritis. He was a lifelong non-smoker.

a. What abnormality can be seen on his chest X-ray?
b. What is the diagnosis?
c. How would you confirm it?

Answers

a. There is a cavitating lesion in the left apex. Also reticulonodular shadowing with upper zone predominance.

b. The most likely diagnosis is reactivation of tuberculosis. Old age and steroids predispose to this. It could be a cavitating lung tumour but this is less likely as he is a non-smoker.

c. Sputum can be sent for smear examination and culture. If he has no sputum then bronchoscopy with bronchial washings may help confirm the diagnosis microscopically. A Mantoux test may be helpful. A positive test indicates previous infection and an exceptionally vigorous reaction suggests current active disease. A Mantoux test has to be interpreted in clinical context.

The patient should be treated with anti-tuberculous drugs even in the absence of microbiological confirmation as clinically the diagnosis is likely. Culture of mycobacterium takes 6 weeks.

Discussion

Tuberculosis is caused by infection with *Mycobacterium tuberculosis*. Other mycobacteria (*M. kansasii, M. xenopi* and *M. avium intracellulare*) can cause pulmonary tuberculosis but these account for the minority of cases. These organisms are particularly resistant to anti-tuberculous therapy. Pathologically the typical appearance of tuberculosis is a caseating granulomatous disease. Macroscopically caseation gives a 'cheesy' appearance.

Pulmonary tuberculosis can be classified into primary, post primary and miliary tuberculosis. Post primary tuberculosis describes the development of tuberculosis a few weeks after the primary infection. It can also represent cases of reinfection or reactivated primary infection in later years. The apicoposterior segments of upper lobes and apical segments of the lower lobes are the most common sites. The patient may present with non-specific symptoms (malaise, weight loss, anorexia), respiratory symptoms (persistent cough, haemoptysis, resistant pneumonia) or there may be no symptoms and the disease is detected on a chest X-ray incidentally. On examination of the chest a variety of physical signs may be found due to collapse, consolidation or even fibrosis. Tuberculosis commonly results in lung fibrosis as this is the result of healing; bronchiectasis is another complication of tuberculosis.

There are a variety of chest X-ray features indicating tuberculosis. The X-ray shown is classical. Other features include:

- Fibrosis (usually apical)
- Hilar gland enlargement, usually unilateral (may resemble bronchial carcinoma) (especially primary TB)
- Miliary shadowing
- Consolidation (often fluffy in appearance)
- Pleural effusion
- Calcification in old lesions (parenchymal and nodal)
- Bronchiectasis and bullae associated with fibrosis.

Treatment with chemotherapy is curative. Quadruple therapy is used at the beginning for 2 months and treatment thereafter continues for 6 months. Close liaison with the microbiologist is essential as resistant strains of mycobacteria are becoming more common.

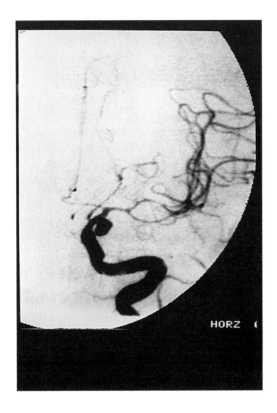

Questions

This patient complained of double vision and a severe headache.

a. What is this investigation?
b. What is the diagnosis?
c. What occular signs may be present (list three)?
d. What is the treatment?

Answers

a. Cerebral arteriogram.

b. An aneurysm of the posterior communicating artery can be seen.

c. Partial ptosis, the eye is fixed in a down and out position (divergent strabismus) and the pupil is dilated (mydriatic). This is a partial third cranial nerve palsy. She has diplopia as she has partial ptosis and this is why it is a partial palsy. The partial ptosis has caused loss of binocular vision to be apparent due to the strabismus and the patient complains of double vision. Clearly this would not be a symptom if the palsy was complete and there was complete ptosis.

d. Clipping of the aneurysm before it ruptures to produce a subarachnoid haemorrhage.

Discussion

An aneurysm of the posterior communicating artery is the commonest cause of a third cranial nerve palsy. If it ruptures to produce a subarachnoid haemorrhage there is associated morbidity and mortality (see Case 57). Other causes of a third nerve palsy include:

- Mid brain vascular lesion
- Demyelinating lesion
- Ophthalmoplegic migraine (recovery is rapid and always complete)
- Neoplastic lesions (carcinoma base of the skull, parasellar neoplasms, meningiomas of the splenoidal wing)
- Mononeuritis multiplex (causes of this include diabetes mellitus, rheumatoid arthritis, polyarteritis nodosa, sarcoidosis, Wegener's granulomatosis, SLE, amyloidosis, carcinomatosis).

A third cranial nerve palsy due to a posterior communicating artery aneurysm never recovers. Intracranial aneurysms account for 75% of cases of non-traumatic subarachnoid haemorrhage. They are found at branching points of arteries, especially around the circle of Willis. The commonest sites are: anterior communicating artery (30%), posterior communicating artery (25%), middle cerebral artery (21%), top of the internal carotid artery (13%), and the posterior circulation (top of the basilar artery and the postero-inferior cerebellar artery). The initial CT scan done for suspected subarachnoid haemorrhage rarely shows the aneurysm and cerebral arteriography is needed prior to surgery.

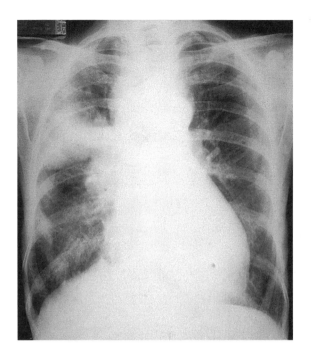

Questions

a. List three abnormalities on this chest X-ray.
b. What is the most likely diagnosis?
c. How would you manage this patient?

Answers

a. There is an enlarged right hilum, mid zone consolidation on the right and a right paratracheal opacity which is probably paratracheal lymph node enlargement.

b. The most likely diagnosis is bronchial carcinoma obstructing the right main bronchus and causing a distal pneumonitis. The right paratracheal lymph node swelling is probably secondary to metastatic disease.

c. The patient should receive treatment for pneumonia (i.e. antibiotics and intravenous fluids, oxygen and bronchodilators as necessary). Bronchoscopy will be necessary for histological diagnosis and also to assess operability. A CT scan of chest will also help with staging. Ipsilateral mediastinal lymphadenopathy is not now considered as necessarily 'inoperable for cure'; however, contralateral lymphadenopathy (N_3) is.

Discussion

Carcinoma of the bronchus can give rise to many clinical manifestations which may be respiratory or symptoms due to metastatic disease, or indeed non-metastatic syndromes (e.g. proximal myopathy, peripheral neuropathy, cerebellar syndrome).

Examining the patient whose chest X-ray is shown may reveal finger clubbing with tar staining of the index finger (not nicotine staining, this is the drug and not the cause of staining). The patient may be cachectic and pale due to anaemia and there may be cervical lymphadenopathy and central cyanosis may be present. There will be reduced expansion on the right side and dullness to percussion in the right mid and upper zones. Bronchial breathing may be heard in the right mid and upper zones over the area of consolidation and there will be increased vocal resonance and whispering pectoriloquy. These are physical signs of consolidation. There is no need to demonstrate tactile vocal fremitus on examination of the respiratory system as this provides the same information as vocal resonance (increased in consolidation, decreased with pleural fluid) and the latter is more sensitive. The patient may have other signs on examination of metastatic disease (e.g. hepatomegaly, skin secondaries).

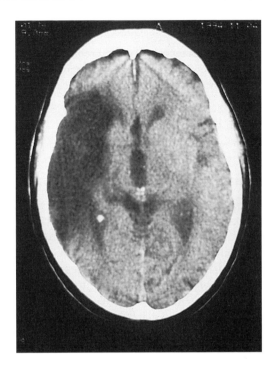

Questions

This 70-year-old man collapsed while shopping. On examination he was deeply unconscious. His routine investigations were as follows:

- Chest X-ray – cardiomegaly
  ECG – left ventricular hypertrophy
- Full blood count normal
- Urea 26.1 mmol/l
- Creatinine 300 mmol/l
- Potassium 5 mmol/l
- Blood sugar 5.6 mmol/l.

a. What does the CT scan show?
b. What is the most likely underlying risk factor?

Answers

a. There is a large right temperoparietal cerebral infarct (black area, a fresh bleed would show up whiter than the brain tissue on a CT scan). This is in the middle cerebral artery distribution.

b. Hypertension is the most likely risk factor. He clearly has long standing hypertension and end organ damage as demonstrated by left ventricular hypertrophy and renal impairment.

Discussion

This patient has had a stroke due to a cerebral infarct. 60% of strokes are due to cerebral infarcts caused by thromboemboli from the carotid or vertebral arteries, 10% of strokes are due to cerebral infarcts from cardiac thromboemboli, 20% of strokes are due to cerebral haemorrhage and 10% of strokes are due to less common causes (e.g. cerebral tumour, abscess, subdural haematoma). There are 100 000 new cases of stroke per year and 80 000 deaths per year from stroke, accounting for 10% of all deaths. Stroke therefore has a high mortality. It also has a significant morbidity in terms of disability. The type of disability depends upon the area of the brain affected. Factors affecting the risk of stroke include: age, family history, hyperlipidaemia, hypertension (increases risk threefold), diabetes mellitus (increases risk twofold), valvular heart disease, ischaemic heart disease (increases risk by threefold), cardiac arrhythmias (non-rheumatic atrial fibrillation increases the risk of stroke by fivefold whereas atrial fibrillation associated with rheumatic mitral stenosis increases the risk by 17-fold).

The patient presented with sudden loss of consciousness and this is an indicator of poor outcome in terms of mortality in the first months. The following are indicators of poor outcome/prognosis:

- Impaired consciousness
- Bilateral extensor plantar response
- Absent pupillary reaction
- Cheyne–Stokes respiration
- Dense paralysis on one side after 1 week
- Sensory impairment
- Urinary incontinence
- Spatial neglect
- Impairment of intellect and memory
- Not walking after 6 weeks.

Whilst the diagnosis is usually obvious clinically CT is of value to distinguish an infarct from haemorrhage. A delay of 3–5 days maximizes detection of infarcts, but they are still often beyond the resolution of CT.

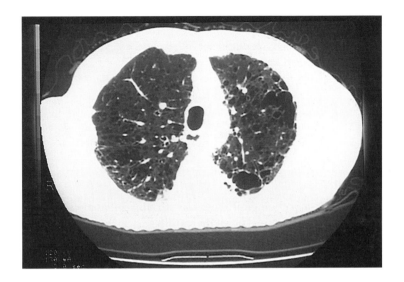

Questions

This 58-year-old smoker complained of a cough and exertional dyspnoea for 5 years. Respiratory function tests showed a reduced vital capacity, increased total lung capacity and residual volume and a reduced transfer factor.

a. What does the CT scan show?
b. What is the diagnosis?
c. What is the treatment?

Answers

a. There is widespread lung destruction (seen as holes) and some bullae (with well defined walls).

b. Emphysema.

c. Stop smoking, bronchodilators, healthy diet, treat intercurrent infection (commonest organisms *Streptococcus pneumoniae* and *Haemophilus influenzae*). Cor pulmonale requires treatment with diuretics.

Discussion

Emphysema is a pathological diagnosis meaning dilatation of the air spaces distal to the terminal bronchioles with destruction of their walls. It is most commonly secondary to cigarette smoking and atmospheric pollution but also is associated with α_1-antitrypsin deficiency. There is clinical overlap with chronic bronchitis which is defined clinically as a productive cough for more than 3 months a year for 3 consecutive years. There are, however, clinical pointers to a diagnosis of emphysema predominating over chronic bronchitis. In emphysema there is marked hyperinflation of the thorax and the patient is usually breathless. There is usually no evidence of central cyanosis and cor pulmonale is a late development. The patient is often described as a 'pink puffer' and is usually undernourished. In chronic bronchitis chest deformity and breathlessness are less common and the patient is usually centrally cyanosed and cor pulmonale is more common. The patient is usually described as a 'blue bloater'. The cachexia associated with emphysema is due to the concomitant breathlessness which deters the patient from eating and also the increased metabolic rate. The chest X-ray can show hyperinflation of the lung fields (the eleventh rib is usually visible) and the hemidiaphragms are flattened with a horizontal pattern of the ribs. Bullae and areas of vascular sparsity are common. The heart shadow is usually long and thin except when heart failure develops which occurs at the end stages. The respiratory function tests show an obstructive pattern as described above. Patients should be tested for reversibility with bronchodilators.

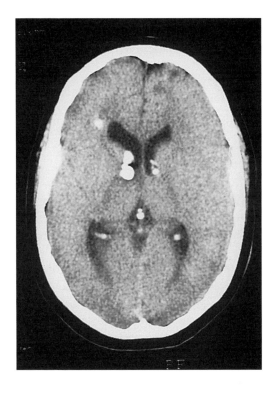

Questions

This is a CT scan of a 27-year-old man who suffers from epilepsy. He also has learning difficulties as does his sister. On examination he has several pink papules on his cheeks and nasal area.

a. What is the abnormality on the CT scan?
b. What is the diagnosis?
c. What is the facial abnormality described?
d. How is this condition inherited?

Answers

a. There are periventricular nodules and calcification.

b. Tuberous sclerosis.

c. Adenoma sebaceum (angiofibromas).

d. Autosomal dominant (25–50% are fresh mutations).

Discussion

Tuberous sclerosis has several names: epiloia, *Bourneville's disease and Pringle's disease. It is a disease which is characterized by a triad of epilepsy, mental retardation and adenoma sebaceum. These last are reddish angiofibromas which develop in childhood on the face, mainly on the cheeks and nasolabial folds. Prevalence of the condition is 5:100 000. There is no treatment other than control of the epilepsy. Clinical features can be categorized as follows:

- Skin. Shagreen patches (circumscribed areas of subepidermal fibrosis occurring in the lumbosacral region), café au lait spots, subungual fibromas, adenoma sebaceum, amelanotic naevi – ovoid depigmented patches on the trunk and limbs which look like a leaf of the mountain ash ('ash leaf melanosis') and are frequently present at birth
- Eyes. Retinal phakomas
- Neurological. Mental retardation, epilepsy, cortical tubers (firm, white areas containing astrocytes and broadening cortical gyri), gliomas, subependymal nodules which calcify, ventricular dilatation
- Skeletal. Bone cysts, sclerotic areas
- Other organs. Cardiac rhabdomyomas, lung and kidney hamartomas.

There is an association with polycystic kidneys and endocrine tumours are common.

---

*D.M. Bourneville (1840–1909), French neurologist.

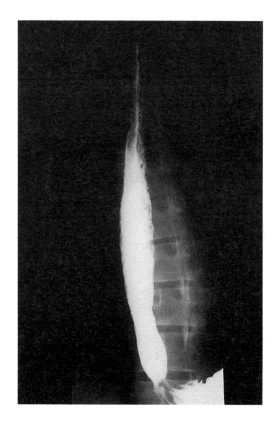

Questions

This 40-year-old man complained of weight loss and pain on swallowing. On examination he had cervical lymphadenopathy and was cachectic. He had extensive areas of his body pierced with gold rings and chains and he had several tatoos.

a. What does his barium meal show?
b. What is the diagnosis?
c. What is the probable underlying diagnosis?

Answers

a. There is irregularity of the oesophagus with ulceration especially in the upper and middle thirds.

b. Oesophageal candidiasis.

c. Acquired immune deficiency syndrome (AIDS).

Discussion

Candidiasis is the most common infection of the oesophagus. It may be an incidental finding on endoscopy or part of a severe systemic infection when the mortality is high. It characteristically occurs in patients who are immunosuppressed and is more common in diabetics. This patient may be immunosuppressed due to malignant disease and his cervical lymphadenopathy may represent secondary infiltration of the lymph nodes or indeed he may have a lymphoma. However, AIDS should be considered, particularly in a patient who clearly has had contact with several needles which may have been contaminated. Oesophageal candidiasis causes pain on swallowing and dysphagia. This is a typical appearance on a barium swallow showing irregularity and ulceration of the oesophageal wall. There is often narrowing of the oesophagus. At endoscopy candidiasis is seen as lumps of white patches on a hyperaemic background of oesphageal mucosa which may be ulcerated in severe cases. The underlying condition should be treated if possible and oesophageal candidiasis is treated with high dose anti-fungal agents given orally (e.g. nystatin).

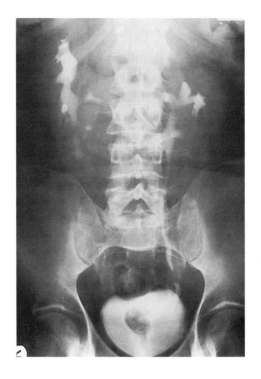

Questions

This patient has had several urinary tract infections.

a. What is this investigation?
b. What does it show?

Answers

a. Intravenous urogram.

b. Horseshoe kidneys.

Discussion

Horseshoe kidneys are a congenital abnormality. The lower poles of the kidneys are fused. Rarely the upper poles may also be fused giving rise to a 'doughnut' deformity. Complications are urinary obstruction, infection and renal stones. The patient may be asymptomatic and the abnormality can be discovered incidentally. Such kidneys are more susceptible to injury.

Radiologically the condition may be visible on plain films with the lower poles of the kidneys being angled more medially than the upper poles (the reverse of the normal situation). On an IVU, as here, the bridge between the kidneys is seen with the characteristic medially-pointing lower pole calyces.

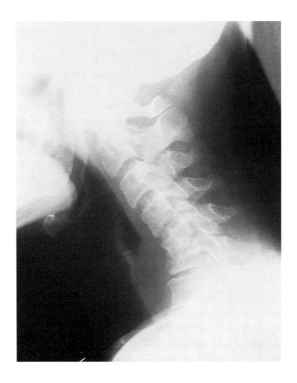

Questions

This is the X-ray of a 70-year-old man who had neck pain and pain in his arms with wasting of the small muscles of the hands. He had had these symptoms for 10 years following a respiratory infection for which he was hospitalized for several months.

a. What does this X-ray show?
b. What is the cause?
c. What was his respiratory infection?

Answers

a. There is destruction of C5/6 vertebral bodies with an angular kyphos ('gibbus') deformity.

b. Old tuberculosis of spine.

c. Pulmonary tuberculosis.

Discussion

Tuberculosis of the spine (*Pott's disease) usually occurs in the lower thoracic/upper lumbar regions but can occur in the cervical region, as in this case, and it tends to start in the vertebral end plate and then spreads to the disc. This is followed by destruction (as shown) if left unrecognized and untreated. Infection can spread along the spine deep to the anterior longitudinal ligament. Patients experience the clinical symptoms of a chronic tuberculous infection (i.e. weight loss, anorexia, malaise) and also experience symptoms localized to the infection (i.e. pain). On examination there is wasting of the associated muscles and a localized kyphos or gibbus deformity with pain on percussion. There is restriction of spinal movements and there may be evidence of cord or root compression. The differential diagnosis includes metastases, myeloma and pyogenic osteomyelitis (commonest organism staphylococcus). Needle or surgical biopsy is needed with culture to confirm the diagnosis. Treatment is with quadruple anti-tuberculous drug therapy and abscesses should be drained. A paraspinal/psoas abscess is common in lumbar disease. The patient should be immobilized and spinal support given until stability is achieved which usually occurs when the vertebral bodies fuse. If the spine is unstable and the cord is at risk then it can be fused surgically.

---

*Percivall Pott (1714–1788). English surgeon.

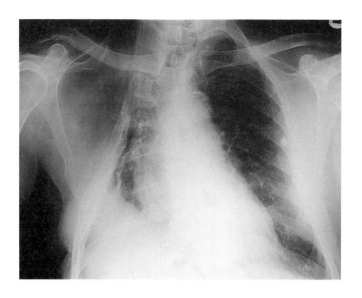

Question

What is the abnormality on this chest X-ray?

Answer

Right thoracoplasty.

Discussion

There is obvious deformity of the chest. This is a thoracoplasty when the upper ribs have been removed surgically (usually the second to fourth ribs). This is an outdated treatment for tuberculosis which was used for this condition prior to the advent of antibiotics. It produced upper lobe collapse and therefore deprived the bacilli of oxygen which they need to thrive in the upper lobes. Other treatments with the same aim were the insertion of foreign materials (e.g. plombage) to create upper lobe collapse. These patients can develop chronic respiratory failure in later life. If this is associated with airways obstruction it is more sinister in these patients as they are unable to produce compensatory overinflation of the lung. Clinically there is obvious deformity of the chest wall with limited movement and a thoracotomy scar is evident. Air entry is reduced and there may be wheezes due to associated airways obstruction or even crackles if pulmonary fibrosis has developed as a consequence of tuberculous infection.

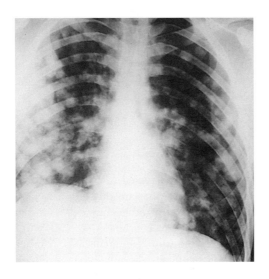

Questions

This 62-year-old man complained of sudden breathlessness. He had had a dry cough for 6 weeks. He also complained of night sweats, polydipsia and headaches. On examination he was breathless and apyrexial, pulse 100 per minute, blood pressure 200/100. Chest auscultation revealed crackles especially on the right side and there was decreased air entry on the left. Investigations were as follows:

- Haemoglobin 18.9 g/dl
- White cell count $11.8 \times 10^9/l$
- ESR 100 mm/hr
- Sodium 126 mmol/l
- Urea 7.8 mmol/l
- Potassium 4.0 mmol/l
- Albumin 30 g/l
- Calcium 2.9 mmol/l
- Random blood sugar 8.1 mmol/l
- Urine – Bence Jones protein negative, blood +++.

a. What is the abnormality on the chest X-ray?
b. What is the most likely underlying diagnosis?
c. Give reasons for the other abnormal tests.

Answers

a. There are multiple lung metastases. These are due to haematogenous spread of a primary tumour. There is also a small left pneumothorax but this is difficult to see on the film; this is the cause of this patient's sudden onset of breathlessness.

b. Adenocarcinoma of kidney also known as a hypernephroma or *Grawitz tumour.

c. Polycythaemia is secondary to a raised erythropoietin secretion by the tumour. Hypercalcaemia (corrected calcium is 3.1 mmol/l) which is causing the symptom of polydipsia is due either to bony secondaries or the production of a parathyroid hormone-like substance by the primary tumour. Hyponatraemia is probably secondary to inappropriate ADH secretion associated with lung metastases. A raised ESR is nonspecific. Microscopic haematuria is one of the presentations of a renal tumour and more commonly there is macroscopic haematuria.

Discussion

The lungs are a common site for metastases. Different sized circular ('coin' or 'cannon ball') lesions can be seen throughout the lung fields due to haematogenous spread of tumour emboli. Tumour emboli are carried to the heart and become lodged in the pulmonary circulation in a random scattered appearance as shown. The commonest tumour to metastasize to lung is lung cancer itself. Other tumours which produce classical cannon ball metastases are: renal, seminoma of testes and osteogenic sarcoma. Secondary deposits in the lungs may cause different chest X-ray appearances apart from the one shown. These include mottling throughout or a solitary metastasis or lymphangitis carcinomatosa. The metastases may cavitate and a lung abscess may form within one or indeed they may rupture and if they are on the periphery a pneumothorax is possible, as in this case.

Adenocarcinoma of the kidneys is more common in males and is usually unilateral. It may be bilateral in 5% of cases. Metastatic spread is usually haematogenous as in the case described but there may be local lymphatic spread and local invasion by the tumour. Clinical presentation is variable and often presentation occurs when the tumour has already metastasized. There may be loin pain, a palpable mass in the loin with micro- or macroscopic haematuria. The patient may complain of episodic fever. There may be evidence of vena caval obstruction or a peripheral neuropathy associated with a tumour. If the tumour spreads into the left renal vein the decreased venous return from the left testis causes a left-sided varicocele as the testicular vein drains into the left renal vein. Endocrine abnormalities may occur as in this case as there is increased erythropoietin production by the tumour and the tumour can also produce parathyroid hormone-like substances and ACTH with consequent clinical features. Hypertension is common. When the diagnosis is suspected an ultrasound scan should be performed which is usually diagnostic showing a mass. An IVU can detect some renal tumours that distort the pelvicalyceal system but it gives less detail and can easily miss even quite a large mass. This should also be accompanied by a CT scan to outline the size and local invasion of the tumour. If there are no metastases, nephrectomy is the treatment of choice and indeed even if metastases are present a nephrectomy can cause regression of the metastases. Solitary metastases may often be worth removing as they represent a single embolic episode. Lymphatic spread of the tumour carries a poor prognosis. If the tumours are bilateral then bilateral nephrectomies and lifelong dialysis may be necessary although sometimes the lesions can be resected and some normal renal tissues conserved. Renal tumours do not respond to chemotherapy or radiotherapy. The overall survival rate is about 50% at 5 years and 30% at 10 years.

---

*P.S. Grawitz (1850–1932). German pathologist.

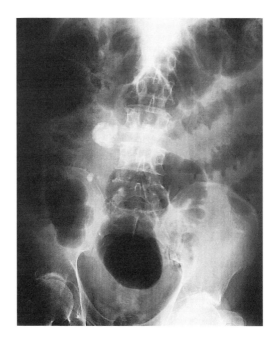

Questions

This 58-year-old man complained of colicky abdominal pain and bloody diarrhoea for 2 days. He had been discharged from hospital 2 weeks previously following a myocardial infarction which was uncomplicated. He was taking aspirin 150 mg daily and atenolol 50 mg daily.

a. What does the abdominal film show?
b. What is the most likely explanation?
c. How should he be managed?

Answers

a. There is a 'thumbprint' appearance on the wall of the small bowel on this plain abdominal film. This can be seen in several conditions including that of small bowel infarction. He has a typical clinical presentation of abdominal pain and bloody diarrhoea.

b. The most likely explanation is that he has developed a left ventricular wall thrombus following his myocardial infarction and thromboembolization has occurred in the mesenteric circulation causing bowel infarction.

c. Initial management should be basic resuscitation as these patients are often very unwell and hypotensive. Blood should be taken for full blood count, electrolytes and cross matching. He should receive intravenous fluids and oxygen as necessary. Small bowel infarction cannot usually be managed conservatively as there is inevitable sepsis and/or perforation if it is left. The patient therefore requires a laparotomy with resection of the infarcted bowel. The patient also requires anticoagulation initially with heparin but this has to be discussed carefully with the surgeon in order to reduce perioperative haemorrhage. Echocardiography is required to confirm the left ventricular thrombus and assess left ventricular function. The patient may have developed a left ventricular aneurysm following his myocardial infarction which may need specific treatment. Mortality for these patients is high.

Discussion

An intracardiac thrombus is more likely to occur following an anterior myocardial infarction and in a dyskinetic segment of myocardium or a left ventricular aneurysm. The complications of a left ventricular thrombus occur when there is thromboembolism which may result in a stroke, mesenteric vascular occlusion, as in this case, or a femoral embolus. The clinical presentations are therefore varied according to which artery/arterial circulation is occluded. Left ventricular aneurysms with or without an intracardiac thrombus also can cause left ventricular failure, ventricular arrhythmias and, rarely, rupture. The confirmation of intracardiac thrombus is best undertaken using transoesophageal echocardiography as transthoracic echocardiography is not sensitive for detecting intracardiac thrombi. If detected, patients require lifelong anticoagulation. Depending on the localization and size of the left ventricular aneurysm an aneurectomy can be performed if significant symptoms are thought probable and the aneurysm is causing significant cardiac decompensation.

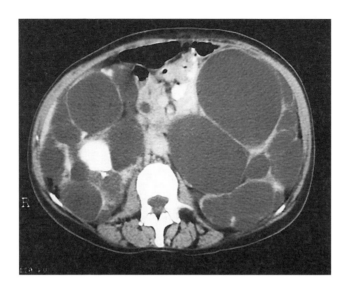

Questions

This is the abdominal CT scan of a 50-year-old woman who presented with a subarachnoid haemorrhage. At presentation fundoscopy revealed papilloedema and haemorrhages and exudates. Her chest X-ray showed cardiomegaly and her ECG revealed a large S wave in V1 and a large R wave in V6. Her maternal aunt had the same condition.

a. What is the abnormality shown?
b. What is the inheritance pattern of this condition?
c. Give reasons for her presentation and the findings described.

Answers

a. Both kidneys are grossly enlarged and occupy most of the abdomen and there are multiple cysts within the kidneys. She has polycystic kidney disease.

b. Autosomal dominant.

c. 60% of cases of polycystic kidney disease are associated with cerebral aneurysms and when these rupture the patient presents with a subarachnoid haemorrhage as in this case. The clinical features described are hypertensive retinopathy (grade IV) and her ECG and chest X-ray confirm she has left ventricular hypertrophy, all of which indicates long standing hypertension. The hypertension is secondary to her renal disease.

Discussion

Adult polycystic kidney disease is common and is inherited as an autosomal dominant condition. The kidneys increase in size gradually as the cysts develop and most cases present in the 3rd or 4th decade. The condition is usually bilateral and rarely unilateral. The patient may present with abdominal pain and distension, recurrent urinary tract infections or the consequences of long standing hypertension. Renal stones may also develop. About 30% of patients also have cysts in the liver which do not usually cause problems and there may be cysts in the pancreas, lungs, spleen and ovaries. As described above, 60% of cases have associated cerebral aneurysms which may rupture producing a subarachnoid haemorrhage which may be the first presentation. As the disease progresses there is chronic renal failure and the patient requires dialysis. These cases are often seen as short cases and the candidate is asked to examine the abdomen. Bilateral masses are easily palpable in the loins but other signs of chronic renal failure should be looked for (i.e. brownish pallor of uraemic anaemia, brown line at the end of the finger nails, bruising, evidence of an AV fistula on the forearm if the patient is undergoing dialysis).

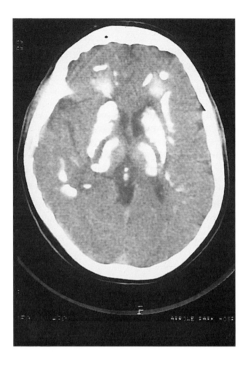

Questions

This 45-year-old woman complained of frequent leg cramps and had developed numbness and paraesthesia in her feet. She complained of increasing tiredness and alopecia and had developed a fungal skin rash. Her investigations revealed the following:

- Electrolytes normal
- Fasting blood sugar 4.1 mmol/l
- Haemoglobin 10 g/dl
- White cell count $2.1 \times 10^9/l$
- Platelets $150 \times 10^9/l$
- MCV 103 fl.

a. What is the abnormality on her CT scan?
b. What is the diagnosis?
c. List two biochemical abnormalities.
d. What is the reason for her leg symptoms?

Answers

a. There is extensive calcification especially in the brain, particularly involving the basal ganglia.

b. Hypoparathyroidism.

c. Hypocalcaemia and hyperphosphataemia. The alkaline phosphatase is normal.

d. Her leg numbness and paraesthesia are due to a peripheral neuropathy which is secondary to the associated pernicious anaemia she has (macrocytic anaemia). Hypoparathyroidism is an autoimmune disease and other autoimmune diseases such as pernicious anaemia are more common. Her leg cramps are secondary to hypocalcaemia.

Discussion

Primary hypoparathyroidism is an autoimmune disease and therefore is associated with other autoimmune diseases which are more common in these patients (e.g. Addison's disease, pernicious anaemia). Hypoparathyroidism may occur following thyroid surgery but usually the surgeon leaves at least one of the four parathyroid glands behind.

The clinical presentation is due to hypocalcaemia which causes paraesthesia (in the extremities and around the mouth) and cramps. Tetany, stridor and convulsions may occur. There is an increased incidence of cataracts and fundoscopy may reveal papilloedema. Cutaneous fungal infections (skin and nails) are common. Calcification in the brain is common. Biochemical abnormalities are a low corrected serum calcium, high serum phosphate and a normal alkaline phosphatase. A plain X-ray of the skull often shows calcification particularly of the basal ganglia.

On examination, as well as the changes described above, the hypocalcaemia will produce positive *Trousseau's and *Chvostek's signs. Trousseau's sign is demonstrated by a sphygmomanometer cuff in which the pressure is elevated to occlude the arterial pulse for 5 minutes. In patients with hypocalcaemia, tetany and carpal spasm will occur (main d'accoucheur). Chvostek's sign is demonstrated by tapping the face over the facial nerve in front of the tragus of the ear. This causes muscular twitching.

The differential diagnosis of hypocalcaemia as well as hypoparathyroidism includes malabsorption, hyperventilation which produces alkalosis, osteomalacia and uraemia. Pseudohypoparathyroidism is an inherited syndrome which occurs in childhood in which the biochemistry is similar to that in idiopathic hypoparathyroidism but there is an inherited failure of the end organ to respond to parathyroid hormone. There is therefore no deficiency of parathyroid hormone but the end organ response is absent. Patients with pseudohypoparathyroidism have a moon face, short stature, learning difficulties and short fourth and fifth metacarpals. To distinguish between hypoparathyroidism and pseudo-hypoparathyroidism the *Ellsworth–*Howard test can be performed. This demonstrates a failure of intravenous parathyroid hormone to cause an increase in urinary phosphate and cyclic AMP excretion.

The treatment of hypoparathyroidism is the treatment of hypocal-caemia and in an emergency this requires intravenous calcium (10 ml with 10% calcium gluconate). In the long term patients require vitamin D and oral calcium supplements.

Basal ganglion calcification is often idiopathic, but its pathological causes include: hypoparathyroidism, pseudohypoparathyroidism, pseu-dopseudohypoparathyroidism, hyperparathyroidism, and lead or carbon monoxide poisoning.

---

*A. Trousseau (1801–1867), French physician.
*F. Chvostek (1835–1884), Austrian surgeon.
*R. M. Ellsworth (1899–1970), American physician.
* J. E. Howard (1902–1985), American physician.

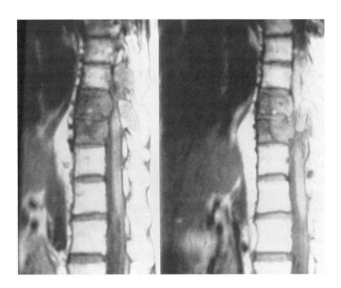

Questions

This 68-year-old man complained of back pain. His investigations revealed the following:

- Raised alkaline phosphatase
- Raised acid phosphatase
- Hypercalcaemia
- ESR 88 mm/hr
- Haemoglobin 10 g/dl
- White cell count $4 \times 10^9/l$
- Platelets $100 \times 10^9/l$.

a. What is the investigation shown?
b. What is the abnormality?
c. What is the most likely underlying cause?

Answers

a. MRI scan of the spine.

b. Metastatic deposits in two of the vertebra which are darker than normal marrow and merge into one another due to local destruction.

c. Metastatic prostatic carcinoma.

Discussion

The biochemical abnormalities in this case point to bony secondaries from a prostatic carcinoma. Serum acid phosphatase, although not used as much nowadays, is almost always raised if there are prostatic secondaries. The pancytopenia may be due to bone marrow involvement and suppression which can occur although it is uncommon.

Prostatic carcinoma is the commonest malignancy in men over the age of 65 years and 20% of cases of prostatic obstruction are due to carcinoma. The tumour may spread locally causing obstruction of one or both ureters or invasion of the rectum resulting in stricture formation. Distant spread by the bloodstream occurs, particularly to bones. Bones most frequently involved are pelvis, vertebrae, upper femur, sternum and skull. Bony metastases from prostate are usually 'sclerotic' or bone forming (osteoblastic) and there may be islands of radiolucency. The usual clinical presentation of bone secondaries is bone pain, pathological fracture or symptoms and signs of hypercalcaemia. The prostate gland can be biopsied transrectally to confirm the diagnosis. In this case bone marrow aspiration is necessary which will also confirm the diagnosis.

Treatment of bony metastases is symptomatic. Bone pain often responds to non-steroidal anti-inflammatory drugs and/or local radiotherapy. Pathological fractures are treated by internal fixation to relieve pain and allow early mobilization. In this case there is spinal cord compression which may require neurosurgical intervention to stabilize the spine. Prostatic tumours have a fairly good prognosis when treated by hormonal manipulation, e.g. oestrogens, orchidectomy. It is worth performing a prostatectomy if there are local symptoms.

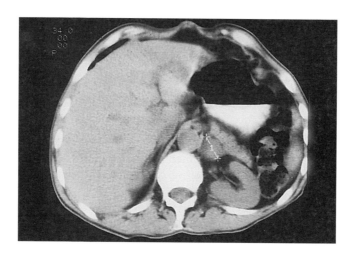

Questions

This is the CT scan of a 68-year-old man who developed increasing areas of pigmentation in the groin and axillae. He complained of increasing breathlessness. On examination he had evidence of a proximal myopathy and there were clinical signs of a left basal consolidation.

a. What abnormality is present on this CT scan?
b. What is the skin lesion described?
c. List two other causes of this skin lesion.
d. What is the underlying diagnosis?
e. What is the reason for his proximal myopathy?

Answers

a. There is a mass anterior to the left kidney (marked) which is a secondary deposit in the left adrenal gland. There is radiographic contrast in the stomach. The liver texture is normal.

b. Acanthosis nigricans. This is a pigmented velvety thickening of the skin which usually occurs in skin folds, most commonly: axilla, groin and sub-mammary areas.

c. Acanthosis nigricans is a cutaneous manifestation of an underlying malignancy most commonly affecting lung, stomach and colon. In the younger age group (less than 40 years) it is usually familial or associated with autoimmune diseases: diabetes mellitus, acromegaly, Addison's disease, hyperthyroidism, hypothyroidism, Cushing's disease, polycystic ovarian disease.

d. Left bronchial carcinoma.

e. His proximal myopathy is one of the non-metastatic manifestations of bronchial carcinoma. Proximal myopathy may occur as part of the syndrome of dermatomyositis which is associated with other underlying malignancies. Other common causes of a proximal myopathy include: osteomalacia, Cushing's disease, iatrogenic steroid excess, thyrotoxicosis.

Discussion

The clinical presentation as described of breathlessness and signs of left basal consolidation along with a proximal myopathy points to an underlying bronchial carcinoma. The adrenal glands are a common site for bronchial metastases. Other sites where bronchial carcinoma typically metastasizes to include: bone, brain, liver and skin. Local spread of a bronchial carcinoma causes symptoms due to the local effect of pressure of the tumour or the enlarged lymph nodes which are metastatic deposits. This can cause superior vena caval obstruction, Horner's syndrome, Pancoast's syndrome, dysphagia, cardiac arrhythmias due to local pericardial spread. Other symptoms and signs depend upon the site of the metastases. However, neuromuscular symptoms can appear as a non-metastatic manifestation of the disease and these include: cerebellar syndrome, peripheral neuropathy, polymyositis, proximal myopathy and myasthenic syndrome. Brain metastases will produce symptoms and signs depending upon their location. The bronchial carcinoma can give rise to other clinical syndromes related to ectopic hormone production which is particularly common with oat cell tumours of the bronchus (ACTH, ADH and prolactin secretion) and squamous cell carcinoma may produce a parathyroid hormone like substance.

CT scanning is a necessary investigation for staging of bronchial carcinoma and detecting metastases. Patients with bronchial carcinoma require a CT scan of the chest and abdomen and may require CT of the brain and an isotope bone scan to detect any metastases. Metastatic disease makes the bronchial carcinoma inoperable. Metastases are not the only cause of adrenal masses. Others include: benign adenoma (may be non-functioning or produce hormonal excess), primary adrenocortical carcinoma, phaeochromocytoma. An adenoma is the commonest though, even in patients with known lung cancer. So an isolated adrenal mass with no other signs of metastases should not be taken as a sign of inoperability of the lung cancer without biopsy of the adrenal mass. Sometimes CT can help to distinguish between these two situations as the high lipid content of adenomas often results in a low CT 'density' reading.

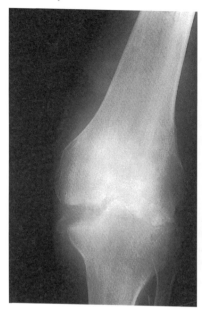
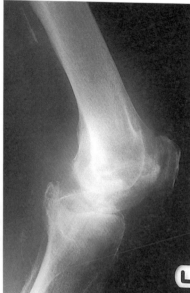

Questions

This patient complained of a painful swollen knee for 4 weeks. He had episodes of shivering and a sore throat 3 weeks previously, after standing on a rusty nail whilst working as a joiner. His general practitioner prescribed flucloxacillin 250 mg qds for 5 days. On examination his temperature was 38°C and he had an effusion on his knee where movement was limited.

a. What does the X-ray show?
b. What is the diagnosis?
c. List the two most important investigations required to confirm your diagnosis.

Answers

a. There is destruction of the articular surfaces with erosions, periosteal reaction and osteopenic areas especially seen in the upper end of the tibia.

b. Septic arthritis.

c. The two most important investigations to confirm the diagnosis are joint aspiration with gram staining and culture of the fluid and blood cultures as he is pyrexial.

Discussion

It is important to diagnose septic arthritis at an early stage to reduce the risk of irreversible joint damage. There is also a mortality associated with this condition if septicaemia develops. *Staphylococcus aureus* is the commonest organism isolated from septic joints. In this case the portal of infection was the rusty nail he stood on a few weeks previously. Other organisms which can produce septic arthritis include: streptococci, pneumococci, gonococci, *E. coli*, pseudomonas and proteus. Septic arthritis may occur without any associated illness, as in this case, but it may be associated with chronic disease such as diabetes mellitus and rheumatoid arthritis when it is more common. It is uncommon to cause septic arthritis following intra-articular injection if an aseptic technique is used. However, joint replacement surgery does increase the risk of sepsis.

Clinically an infected joint is swollen, tender and hot and there is muscle spasm. Usually a single joint is infected but there may be more than one. There is local lymphadenopathy and systemic upset with malaise, fever, rigors, nausea and vomiting. Diagnostic difficulties sometimes delay diagnosis when there is infection in an abnormal joint, particularly rheumatoid arthritis. If the diagnosis is suspected joint aspiration should be performed immediately with the joint drained to dryness and the synovial fluid sent for gram staining and culture. It is important to search for a source of infection (e.g. infected skin lesions, boils, recent respiratory or genitourinary infections). Blood cultures should always be taken as they are sometimes helpful when the synovial fluid has failed to provide any significant microbial growth. In the early stages the plain X-ray of the joint is normal (unless there is underlying arthritis of course) and if the diagnosis is delayed then joint destruction as described above occurs. This progresses to osteomyelitis which produces the osteopenic appearance, as in the tibia in this case. The differential diagnosis includes gout, pseudo gout, acute rheumatoid arthritis or seronegative arthritis but in all these conditions the joint fluid is sterile.

Treatment consists of bed rest with immobilization of the joint and joint aspiration to dryness to remove pus and relieve pain. Repeated re-aspirations are usually necessary to remove reaccumulated pus. Surgical intervention is almost never required. Broad spectrum antibiotics should be given initially and as *S. aureus* is the commonest organism the anti-biotics should be effective against this. Intravenous antibiotics may be required in the first few days if the patient is very ill and then they can be prescribed orally for a period of at least 6 weeks. Other treatment should include analgesics and also physiotherapy to prevent muscle wasting and joint deformity. The prognosis depends upon how soon the diagnosis is made and treatment commenced. If treatment is commenced before any joint damage has occurred the outlook is good but infection of the hip joint in children and all infections in the elderly have a poorer prognosis. Patients with rheumatoid arthritis also have a poorer prognosis, mainly due to the associated delay in diagnosis as the symptoms and signs are erroneously thought to be due to a flare-up of rheumatoid disease.

Index